HORMONE OPTIMIZATION

Unlock Your Innate Ability to Burn Fat, Build Muscle and Feel Unstoppable

Joonas Virtanen

ISBN: 9798607645014

Cover design by: Drey Creative
Library of Congress Control Number: 2018675309
Printed in the United States of America

CONTENTS

Title Page

Copyright

Introduction   1

Chapter 1: The basics   7

The second most complex system ever observed   8

Chapter 2: Health   16

First things first: Health   17

Chapter 2.1 Sleep   19

Sleep is the most important thing in your life   20

What influences sleep quality   24

Chapter 2.2 Gut health   28

Humans are animals   29

Eating and not eating   32

Food is fuel   35

Food is nutrition   38

Absorbing food   41

Food is also feeding your gut bacteria   43

Chapter 2.3 Stress   47

Addicted to stress   48

The autonomic nervous system   51

Staying social   56

Chapter 2.4 Movement — 58

Your brain moves you — 59

Avoiding aches and pains — 60

To cardio or not to cardio — 64

Exercise motivation — 69

Minimum effective dose — 72

Working out and working in — 73

Chapter 3: Losing Weight — 75

Weight Loss — 76

Losing weight or losing fat? — 79

Calories in, calories out — 82

Different energy systems of the body — 85

Correct hormonal environment can make all the difference — 88

The impact of different hormones — 94

Lifestyle practices for optimal hormonal function — 102

What about supplements? — 106

Hacks and tweaks — 107

Closing words — 112

Chapter 4: Gaining Strength and Muscle — 114

Bodybuilding? — 115

Muscle and strength 101 — 117

Wait, did you just call me a newbie? — 120

Training the central nervous system strength — 122

Training for bigger gas tanks within the muscles — 125

Training for bigger engines within the muscles — 127

Fueling your training — 130

Training regimen for optimal hormone balance — 135

Rest, recovery and tracking ... 141

Getting shredded ... 143

But I just want to look like Brad Pitt in Fight Club ... 146

Cheat days and letting loose ... 148

Lifestyle habits for correct hormonal balance ... 150

Supplements ... 151

Tips and troubleshooting ... 153

Closing words ... 157

Chapter 5: Resources and Recommendations ... 158

INTRODUCTION

Want to get into better shape? You can forget about starving yourself or going full beast-mode at the gym 7 days a week. This book will explain how you can easily create dramatic body composition changes by optimizing your own natural hormones. And the best part is that what's going to make you look better is also going to make you feel and perform better. It's important to understand that hormones don't exist in a vacuum. They are a part of a larger whole. But hormones are a great shorthand for talking about all the things that need to happen for you to achieve specific health and fitness outcomes. There aren't any obese men in the world who also have a high testosterone and have a well-functioning insulin system. Correlation does not equal causation, but it doesn't really matter in this case. If you practice lifestyle habits that target raising your testosterone and keeping your insulin in check, you are on the right path towards weight loss and muscle building. And that's why hormones are useful. Think of them as signposts on your way to your goals. Weight loss and muscle gain are simply emergent side effects of having the correct hormone balance in the body.

Even though hormones aren't the whole story, they alone can be massively powerful. Take a moment to think about anabolic steroids in sports. The reason they are banned is literally because they work too well. They are deemed unfair to competition because they produce such insane results, making their users stronger, bigger and shredded. Now here's the kicker: Anabolic steroids are hormones. Same stuff your body makes.

There's a study where a group of healthy men were divided into three groups: those who exercised, those who exercised and used anabolic steroids and those who only took anabolic steroids but didn't exercise. The group who only took steroids, but didn't exercise, built more muscle than the group who only exercised! Of course I'm not telling you to go out and inject yourself full of synthetic hormones, but rather optimize your own innate production of these supernatural strength builders and fat burners.

Not convinced yet? Here's one last example: Teenagers. What happens to kids when they become teenagers? Girls grow more fat in all the right places, guys tend to get skinnier but more muscular. Did these kids suddenly start working out and eating healthy? No, quite the opposite actually. But the natural shift in hormone production changes their bodies even if the environmental factors aren't favorable. That's how powerful hormones can be.

Regardless of your goals (more muscle, less fat, more energy, better health), being mindful of hormones first is a very powerful strategy. When you start looking at things like diet, exercise, sleep, mindfulness (and all the other buzzwords the health industry throws around) in the light of what they do to your hormones, the story starts to make a lot more sense. You don't need to question if you should be doing this or that, or whether this vegan cupcake will make you fat. You'll know how these different things will impact you because you'll know what they do to your hormone balance. And suddenly losing weight, getting strong and healthy becomes way less stressful. You'll have a systematic approach that makes sense. One that will still allow you to enjoy the things you love the most. I don't care if you're a vegan female or a carnivore male, the same fundamental principles will still apply.

P.S. Even if your goal is to build bigger muscles, you should still read the chapter regarding weight loss first. And if your goal is weight loss, definitely don't skip the muscle building chapter right after. Both of these concepts are very much interlinked and the hormonal dynamics at play are similar. Simply put, both will benefit each other.

Study link:

https://www.ncbi.nlm.nih.gov/pubmed/8637535

I'm not a fitness celebrity or a doctor. I was a combat medic in the Finnish military, but in all honesty that really just means that I can put together a really nice cast out of twigs. I'm just a guy who's worked his whole career in advertising and marketing, who ran into some pretty serious health issues around 2012 and had to learn to take his health into his own hands. Luckily the marketing background is actually a pretty good fit here. The reason why companies hire people to help out with their marketing is because the companies are too deep in the trenches to see the world around them. Successful advertising and marketing people become experts at understanding what the problem is and how to fix it. This requires looking at the bigger picture, identifying the company's blindspots and addressing them. The entire health/wellness/fitness space seems to be struggling with this same problem. It's siloed, with different groups in their own foxholes, telling you to go vegan, go keto, go running, lift weights, do yoga, all the while blind to the big picture. People are different and no single approach is going to apply to everyone.

It's also good to know that even though there are thousands and thousands of experts in the world of health and wellness, they often don't see eye to eye. There's a lot of stuff about human physiology we simply don't understand yet. That's why I'm going to focus on the things we do know and stay away from the esoteric or theoretical debates. The value I bring to the discussion is in synthesizing information from a variety of sources and wrapping it in a package that's fairly easy to understand without a doctor's degree.

But back to my story: I had a problem and I had to solve it. Nobody else was going to do it for me. Believe me, I tried that approach first. Doctors tested everything they could, nothing worked. I'll get into more detail later in this book but my health problem was gut-related. So I dove deep into the world of gut health experts, and with each step a thousand more paths opened up before me. Should I try gluten-free? Should I try paleo? Or maybe keto? Are carbs good or are they bad? What macros should I eat? What are macros? You get the idea.

Over the years I spent tens of thousands of hours and an equal amount of dollars trying to understand what was wrong and how can I fix it. I studied, I tried things, fasted for days, bought every supplement known to man, I did expensive lab testing, you name it. Eventually my body of knowledge on knowledge of the body got quite good. Excuse the pun. After I fixed my own gut issues and got healthy again, I got interested in optimizing my function further and wound up taking my personal fitness to a whole new level. Getting stronger and shredded was and is fun, but it's also a pretty selfish endeavor.

And that brings me to why I wanted to write this book. After being so caught up in the health and fitness space for years it started to feel like I could see the code behind the Matrix and felt frustrated. All these "experts" arguing about such meaningless points when in reality there are a few simple lifestyle modifications everyone should be focusing on first. And those things all involve managing your hormones. It also just so happens that the same interventions that are good for fat burning and muscle building also happen to be the most powerful tools to improve brain health, gut health and on it goes.

I did all that heavy lifting in figuring this stuff out so you don't have to. But if you are very interested in geeking out and diving deep, this book can serve as a good launching pad on a variety of subjects. However, you'll need to look for the nitty gritty stuff elsewhere. I simply want to share my framework with you and hopefully teach you that you don't need to understand every little detail of everything. To get big results, lift the big rocks first. That's what this book focuses on: the big rocks of health, wellness, muscle building and fat burning.

CHAPTER 1:
THE BASICS

THE SECOND MOST COMPLEX SYSTEM EVER OBSERVED

The human brain wins this one. But a close second is mammalian metabolism. The system that drives life inside of you. The system that will make you fat, skinny, strong, weak, anything you tell it to do.

I'm a fan of analogies. Imagine the human body as a very complicated weird factory, like something straight out of a steampunk book. You pull a lever here and this liquid gets poured into a cup here which tilts the balance of the cup, kipping it over, liquid dripping down a conveyor belt which is moving straight into an oven, hardening the liquid to little crystals which in turn are dumped into another bowl of liquid. The reaction between the crystals and the liquid causes gas to form, the gas then rises up, filling a balloon which eventually takes off, hits a switch in the ceiling which opens a door to a cage where weird critters crawl out of and on it goes. What the hell am I talking about?

See if I described the metabolic machinery in your body, it would sound equally strange and complicated. Nothing happens in isolation, everything is interconnected and insanely complex. As one example: here's a snapshot of the Krebs cycle in someone whose body is not that great at making energy on a cellular level:

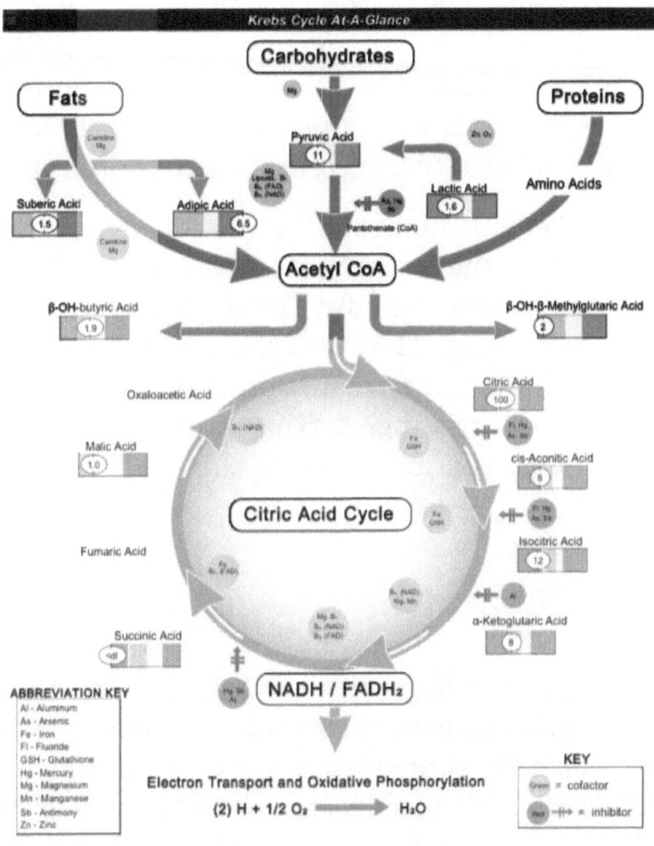

Pretty simple to fix it right? Just improve your conversion of fats into suberic and adipic acid, get better at converting carbs into pyruvic acid and proteins into amino acids to create more Acetyle CoA, then improve the steps along the way to create more citric acid which in turn creates cis-Aconitic Acid which again turns into isocitric Acid and so it goes into eternity. By the way, that is a snapshot of my own Krebs cycle back in the day. Clearly I had some issues making ATP and fueling the biology of life inside of me. Since then things have improved quite a bit. But I digress.

Krebs cycle is one example of the millions of complicated

chemical experiments going on in your body at all times. Together they form a system that is stronger together than any individual part alone. The reason why humans are very resilient animals is because there is a lot of redundancy built into the system. If one part fails, it never crashes the whole system. But over time the factory, that is you, starts to operate less and less efficiently if you keep steering it in the wrong direction.

And this is where hormones come in. Think of hormones as the workers operating the imagery factory. They don't create the liquids or the crystals, the bowls or the balloons, they simply operate the machinery. They pull the levers so to speak. They tell your body, the factory, what to do at any given time. Should we be growing or shrinking? Getting stronger or leaner? Is this a life-threatening situation or are we safe? Let's introduce those workers:

Testosterone

We are all pretty familiar with testosterone. It's the primary male hormone. It can make us stronger, more aggressive, more driven and generally more masculine. Give too much to a man and he might be a bit too aggressive and assertive. Too little and you'll get a depressed unmotivated weakling. Too much in a woman and you end up with masculine bodily features (facial hair, lowered voice, etc). Too little in a woman and again you get someone who has a very hard time getting anything done. It's worth noting that testosterone raising advice in this book won't make any woman unnaturally masculine.

Testosterone is often used (illegally) as a performance enhancing supplement and the reason is quite clear: High levels will make any human stronger. That's why testosterone is your best friend when it comes to building muscle and burning fat.

With age the testosterone levels in both men and women tend

to diminish. On top of that, average testosterone numbers around the world in men have been dropping like crazy over the last 30 years. The reason isn't 100% clear but obesity definitely plays a part. Other contributing suspected causes include pollution and increased use of plastic. Certain compounds in plastics are known as xenoestrogens, meaning they can mimic estrogen. This increased estrogenic activity will then drive testosterone down in the body, as the hypothesis goes.

Estrogen

Estrogen is basically the yin to testosterone's yang. It's the primary female hormone, responsible for feminine feature development in the body. Where the ratio of testosterone to estrogen in men is high, it's lower in women. Any healthy person is going to have both at all times but the ratios differ. Estrogen levels play a huge role in women on multiple levels, regulating basically everything to do with fertility. Estrogen isn't covered much in the book simply because it's not as straightforward and actionable when it comes to fat burning or muscle building, as the other ones. Very likely the actions you take to balance other hormones will also have a positive effect towards estrogen.

As with testosterone, with age estrogen levels in women tend to drop.

Insulin

Again, a pretty familiar term to most people mostly due to extremely high diabetes numbers around the world. As I'm sure you know, diabetes is essentially a condition where the body needs additional insulin to regulate blood sugar. Insulin regulates energy intake from carbs, fats and protein. It also regulates growth quite a bit. High insulin levels will create bigger mammals which is why bodybuilders have been messing with insulin for a long time. Strategic use of insulin can indeed help out with muscle building but it can also kill you if you're not careful.

Insulin levels and utilization within the body can be skewed over time by unhealthy diet and lifestyle. Insulin-resistance is a commonly recognized state where the body is "numb" to insulin. It's been flooded with insulin for so long that the system slowly stops working. The end result of this process is Type 2 Diabetes.

Human Growth Hormone

The ultimate Mr Fix-It of the body. Human Growth Hormone or HGH is responsible for repair and growth of pretty much anything in the body. HGH is not only important for muscle growth, it's fundamental to the body on a cellular level. HGH is also very often used as a performance enhancer in sports, mainly because it can speed up recovery like nothing else.

HGH (or lack of it) plays a crucial role in how body fat is stored. Supplemental HGH has been shown to reduce visceral fat, which is unhealthy and aesthetically the most unpleasant form of body fat. HGH deficiency will lead to increased visceral fat.

Over time the HGH levels will decline and one of the more common "anti-aging" strategies is actually to give elderly people human growth hormone.

Cortisol

Cortisol gets a lot of press these days. It's the STRESS HORMONE, which sounds pretty bad. But cortisol is also vital: It wakes you up in the morning and is actually a pretty powerful fat burner on it's own. As with every other hormone, it's all about balance.

Even though cortisol resistance is not being talked about (yet?),

I would argue that there's a similar story cooking here as with insulin. If you flood your body with cortisol all the time, you'll need more and more of it to get the same results and eventually you become numb to its effects.

Dopamine

The motivation hormone, also known as the addiction hormone. Most pleasurable things in life will spike dopamine and so do the most addictive drugs and vices.

And again, dopamine resistance is a real thing. Spike dopamine all the time and smaller peaks don't feel like anything anymore. This phenomenon helps explain why extreme athletes need crazier and crazier challenges to get their fix, but it's also a likely culprit in the modern depression epidemic. The modern environment is full of dopamine triggers and over time we become more and more numb to its effects. Without dopamine, everything in life feels grey and meaningless. Easy to see how that could lead to a deep depression.

Melatonin

Melatonin makes you sleepy. Pretty simple. If you're not making enough melatonin you're not getting good sleep and resting properly. Make too much of it at the wrong time and get sleepy when you shouldn't. But melatonin is also crucial for the other hormones to work properly. Not enough melatonin means your sleep isn't up to par and you're not making enough HGH and testosterone.

Vitamin D

Vitamin D is actually a hormone, not a vitamin. And not

only that, it's the wakefulness hormone to counter melatonin's sleepy qualities. It is crucial to a host of things processes inside the body, and again the right amount is crucial. Ideally we make vitamin D from sun exposure, but people living in the northern parts of the world, such as myself, need to be supplementing over the winter months to sustain adequate levels.

Leptin And Ghrelin

The hormone leptin is intricately involved in the regulation of appetite, metabolism and calorie burning. Leptin is essentially a satiety hormone. It's the chemical that tells your brain when you're full and when it should start burning up calories.

The purpose of ghrelin is basically the exact opposite of leptin: It tells your brain when you need to eat, when it should stop burning calories and when it should store energy as fat.

Dysregulation of these two hormones can lead to overeating and obviously plays a huge part in the modern obesity epidemic.

Other Hormones: Igf-1, Dhea, Progesterone, Thyroid Hormone, Estradiols...

Now there are a LOT of different hormones in the body and the reason we're not going to dive deep into each one of them is because they simply aren't as actionable as the ones mentioned above. The point of this book is not to explain the ins and outs of every hormone in your body but rather teach you to look at things in the context of the hormones that are important to your health goals.

Hormones Are Feelings

Hormones aren't just powerful signaling molecules, they also evoke feelings. Thinking happens via electric impulses in the brain. Feelings on the other hand, happen chemically.

Feeling stressed raises cortisol. But elevating cortisol also induces the feeling of heightened awareness or anxiety, essentially stress. Testosterone makes you feel strong. But even winning in something non-physical like a poker game will raise your testosterone. Growth hormone makes you feel more energetic, and things that make you feel more energetic tend to raise growth hormone. Dopamine makes you more motivated, and thus motivational things will elevate dopamine. And don't get me started on leptin and ghrelin which heavily influence your eating habits.

Managing your hormones is then also about managing your emotions. And the right hormone balance will create the right emotional balance. This is maybe the biggest reason why I think it's so good to focus on hormones when it comes to hitting your health and fitness goals. This approach guarantees that your path towards your goals will feel good and rewarding, not just in a theoretical sense, but in a very real emotional way.

CHAPTER 2: HEALTH

FIRST THINGS FIRST: HEALTH

Before we jump into specifics of losing weight or gaining muscle, it's important to make one thing clear: If you're not healthy, you're making things a whole lot more difficult for yourself. Of course health is an insanely vague term. But if you remember the analogy about lifting the big rocks first, we can use the same approach here. Lift the big rocks when it comes to health and you're pretty much checking all the boxes that matter.

We in the West tend to think of health as the absence of illness and while there is some truth to that, your body doesn't really "think" about health the same way. You're a system that is either in balance or not. Minor imbalances might not result in a visible illness but over time the system will tilt more and more towards chaos that will cause problems.

Dr Terry Wahls, who has basically cured her own multiple sclerosis with an ancestral paleo diet, has a great saying: The best way to fight disease is to create health. And I wholeheartedly agree with this approach. Instead of trying to figure out an antidote or a magic bullet to fight a health problem, aim to create more health within the body and allow the system to take care of the problems. Your body is smarter than you. Trust it.

Look back to the factory analogy. If things are going haywire would the best approach to fixing it really be throwing a wrench (or a pill) into the machinery? Sure it will change something about the process that is happening but you're not taking it any closer to achieving equilibrium

So with this systems approach in mind, how do we go about creating health? Or to put in another way, what are the big rocks we need to lift first? The foundational pillars of health are as follows:

1) Good sleep
2) Excellent gut health
3) Balanced stress levels
4) Empowering movement

CHAPTER 2.1 SLEEP

SLEEP IS THE MOST IMPORTANT THING IN YOUR LIFE

Sleep is fundamental to any organism. It's good to take a minute to appreciate just how important sleep actually is. Evolutionarily sleep doesn't really make any sense: why would any organism do something that leaves them completely vulnerable to prey one third of their whole life? If sleep wasn't absolutely critical, animals (including humans) that slept would've disappeared a long time ago, outcompeted by their brethren that don't need to sleep. But we all sleep.

The reason why sleep is on top of this list isn't only the evolutionary background. It's because today's culture is an enemy of sleep on so many levels. We idolize the tech start-up entrepreneur who spends his nights coding and drinking coke. We are also drowning in new Netflix shows to watch, new video games to play, new night clubs to try out, endless things to keep you up at night. There's a fairly new word that had to be invented to describe a problem that never used to exist: social jetlag. That's when you shift your schedule every weekend a few hours ahead and then spend the majority of the week recovering from this self-induced jetlag simply to do it all over again the following weekend. The term is derived from going out socially but I would argue the problem is probably even more commonly caused by binge watching TV or staying up in front of the computer or smartphone.

Quantifying "Good Sleep"

So how much sleep should you be getting? Everyone knows the answer: 8 hours. But within this truth lies a dangerous misconception. Not all sleep is created equal. You can sleep for 8 hours and wake up feeling absolutely miserable or sleep for 6 and bounce up full of energy. It's the quality of the sleep that matters way more than the amount. Technology has pretty much ruined our sleep in the last 10 years so it's only fair that technology is making up for this mistake. It's now easier than ever to actually measure your sleep to get an idea of how well you are resting. Almost any wearable fitness device includes some sort of sleep tracking nowadays and one of the best in the bunch in 2020 is called the Oura Ring. I personally use the Oura Ring so the following examples will be based on that, but most likely any fairly modern fitness tracker will do a decent job of quantifying your sleep.

To explain what comprises a night of sleep, let's take a look at this image from the Oura app:

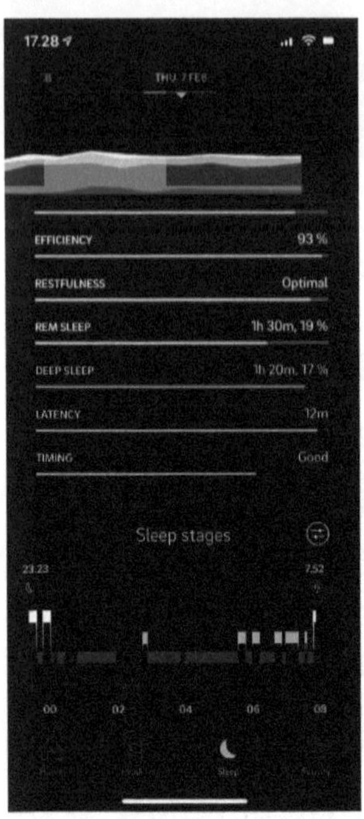

White bars represent being awake, light bar is REM sleep, medium bar is light sleep and darkest bar equals deep sleep.

The key things to focus on are the amount of REM sleep and deep sleep. You can find tons of info on the importance of REM sleep online with a simple Google search but since we'll be focusing on hormonal health we should be looking at deep sleep specifically. Deep sleep is probably the most important single marker that will contribute to good hormone health. You should be getting at least 1-2h of deep sleep per night but this will vary individually. Deep sleep also tends to decrease as we age and according to research, and an 80 year old is only getting 5% of the deep sleep they got when they were young.

As you can see from the image, and what studies also show, most deep sleep occurs early in the night. For myself personally it's always between 11pm and 4am. REM sleep on the other hand comes into play later in the night, or early in the morning. If you go to bed very late, you will lose deep sleep because you can't simply make up for those early night hours by waking up later. You will get more REM sleep with this strategy but not more deep sleep. Remember the term social jetlag? The reason that jetlag happens is that your body's "internal clock", also known as the circadian clock, is set a certain way and it will take several days/nights to shift it back and forth. Your body's machinery is used to running certain operations at specific times and it will always try to do that first. If you simply stay up late one day, your body will not automatically switch into this new rhythm and thus you will sacrifice on sleep quality. You should always try to go to bed around the same time and wake up around the same time. In the context of modern life it's not always possible so make it a priority whenever you can.

Study links:

ttps://www.ncbi.nlm.nih.gov/pmc/articles/PMC3142094/

https://www.medicalnewstoday.com/articles/324640

WHAT INFLUENCES SLEEP QUALITY

So a steady circadian rhythm is important for sleep quality. Got it. What else will affect it? Alcohol is a huge one. Even a couple of drinks will raise your heart rate, body temperature and cause you to get less deep sleep. Similarly, exercising too late in the evening can be very bad for sleep. It takes time for your body to wind down and enter into that restful parasympathetic state (more on that later) and late-night workouts will shift your circadian rhythm forward.

Even if you're not exercising too late in the evening, simply exercising too hard or too much can wreck your sleep. One of the biggest benefits about sleep tracking to me personally has been the connection between working out and sleep. I used to think that the harder I can train the better and then I'll just rest even harder to balance it all out. Doesn't work like that. When I cut down on the volume and intensity of my workouts, I started to sleep better. Better sleep leads to better hormonal balance which leads to better recovery which leads to more strength and muscle. Ironically by working out less, I was getting more results. More on exercise strategies in the later chapters.

Stress in general is probably the most common reason for sleep issues in modern times. The big thing to keep in mind is that all stress is stress. If you're stressed at work and stressed at home, stressing yourself more at the gym isn't going to help. And you definitely can't sleep your way out of stress because stress will wreck your sleep. It can be a very vicious cycle and not something to be taken lightly. You should try to come up with a personal de-stressing routine before you go to bed. And it doesn't need to be anything spiritual and woowoo. Simply reading a book or even watching Netflix for a couple of hours on the couch (not in bed) is way better than running around the house. As long as it's not a horror show. But keep the electronics out of your bedroom. More on stress management in the following chapters.

Diet and sleep are also strongly interlinked but since we'll be focusing on the big rocks and not the nitty-gritty, there's one big rule when it comes to food and sleep: Don't eat too late. You should always allow at least 2 hours between your last meal and going to sleep. The reason why this is beneficial is that allows your body to handle the heavy lifting of digesting food first so it can focus on sleeping and repairing when the time comes. Another easy tip to keep in mind is that you shouldn't go to bed feeling hungry or stuffed. So your last meal should be something balanced and large enough to keep hunger away for a few hours but not a massive undertaking that will take your body hours to digest.

Managing your light exposure is one of the best ways to influence your circadian rhythm. You'll want to get plenty of bright light in the day, starting as early in the morning as possible, and you'll want to avoid bright light at night. Again, this is an area where you can go crazy and only live by candlelight in the evenings but there's no need to go overboard. There are a couple of no-brainers that everyone should pay attention to though:

1)   Reducing Blue Light At Night

If you need to look at a screen late in the evening, be it a cellphone, laptop or TV, you can reduce the light impact by installing a software that will turn the screen yellowish red. Basically you're taking away most of the blue light emitted by the screen.

This is important because blue light wavelengths are the primary ones that signal to your brain that it's daytime. Clear blue skies aren't a signal to go to bed, right? Blue light is also rougher on the eyes than other forms of light and most prescription glasses now come with an option to get them with a coating that reduces blue light exposure. I've got a pair like that. I wear contacts during the day time but at night I've always got my glasses on which will further reduce the blue light exposure.

If you got a laptop, install software called f.lux or use the operating system settings to reduce the blue light a few hours before going to bed. Same with your cell phone and any other electronic device with a screen. Another useful tip is to install a couple of dim night lights to your house so you don't need to turn all the lights on every time you go to the bathroom late at night. Darkness is a very clear and powerful signal for your body to start making melatonin, the sleep hormone. More melatonin, more restful uninterrupted sleep.

2) Getting Plenty Of Bright Light During The Day

If the sun has risen when you wake up, go out for at least 15 minutes early in the day. If the sun has not risen yet, turn on all the lights you have at your house. If you got a bright light device (pretty common item in the northern countries), use it. The most important light exposure for anchoring your rhythm happens in the morning, but it's still useful to go out regularly during the day. No matter how bright your office lamps are, they don't compare to the sun. If your desk is next to a window and your office has really bright lighting, you're getting roughly 1000 lux worth of light to your eyes. This is not bad, but being out in the sunlight you'd be getting 10 000 lux. Not to mention the fact that mostly you're not going to be hanging out next to a window so in reality you're probably getting some hundred lux throughout the day. Our eyes are "calibrated" for light levels of

1000 - 10000 lux during the day. Anything less than that means it's night time in the natural world. Be mindful of your light exposure.

Summary:

- Quality over quantity
- Deep sleep is the most important sleep marker
- Steady circadian rhythm is key in promoting healthful sleep cycles
- Stress, especially late in the evening wrecks your sleep
- Leave at least a 2 hour gap between your last meal and going to bed
- Manage your light exposure: dark at night, plenty of light during the day

CHAPTER 2.2
GUT HEALTH

HUMANS ARE ANIMALS

As an introduction to the chapter relating to gut health, I think it's important to consider the human as an animal like any other. Human diet is such a hotly debated issue in society, but nobody even bothers to debate whether it's a good idea to feed zoo animals the kinds of foods they are used to in the wild. It just feels obvious, right? So why are we humans so confused about what we should eat? Because there are no "wild" humans left we could use as reference. I mean there are some uncontacted tribes left in the Amazon and a couple of other spots but their diet doesn't seem like a realistic reference to someone living in the Northern part of the globe. So the point is sort of moot.

But there is an obvious answer to this debate: People should mainly eat how their ancestors ate. That's the closest to a modern "zoo human" eating like the wild human ate. The real debate then becomes how far back we should look. Should I eat like my grandma? Or my great great great grandma? Go far enough into history and we're all Africans. There are no 100% answers to be found in this area for a very long time, but as a guiding principle this ancestral way of thinking is very solid. It may not seem "fair" that you should be forced to eat what everyone around you has always eaten but nature isn't fair. Here's a concrete example: Most people in the world are lactose intolerant. They simply can't digest lactose because their ancestors never needed to. They had no cows, so after breastfeeding was over, the body never saw another lactose molecule. Lactose tolerance on the other hand is only common in Northern Europe and in people whose ancestors originate from that area, because cattle farming was so prevalent. The DNA mutation which allows a person to consume lactose was great for survival. So over millennia and millennia the milk consuming populations did better than the rest. And the end result is that most of the population in Northern Europe can digest lactose. We in Northern Europe actually diagnose lactose intolerance as a condition that one is suffering from when in reality the people who can digest lactose are the weird ones. So let's say you're Chinese and really love milk. You are forever doomed to lactose-free varieties or suffering the consequences: gut distress, bloating, etc. Not fair, just biology. Now the lactose example is an easy one because it's so simple: change one enzyme, one DNA strain and boom, no problem. But you could apply the same thinking to any other food item or way of eating. If your ancestors never encountered this type of diet, you probably aren't very well suited for it. And there's one thing we do know for sure: Nobody in your family tree ever ate the kind of diet that is pushed to us by modern food marketers every day. Thus, nobody in modern society is adapted to eating a 'high sugar high processed fast food' diet. Nobody.

Animals can also give interesting clues to how prehistoric humans might have behaved. For example my dog could care less about a piece of candy but goes crazy over raw liver or fish. Would be interesting if you could ask a prehistoric human if their palate worked in a similar way. The dog clearly values potential nutritional value of food over high sugar content whereas us modern humans only tend to think about the taste of food. *I like this, I don't like that.* But taste is just one aspect of food. Some foods don't taste that good but provide tons of nutrition. Other foods taste amazing but are empty inside. And some obviously do both. But every piece of food has both immediate and long term consequences. We often recognize that we're not going to feel very good after eating something "bad" such as cake. But for a few fleeting seconds of mouth pleasure we're often willing to overlook these consequences.

I tend to think that somewhere along the way we lost the ability to sense these other aspects of food. Everything we eat tastes good and we've become numb to everything else. Every wild animal intuitively knows what foods they should eat and when. Grazing cows for example tend to eat different varieties of grass at different times for no apparent reason, before you take a closer look at their biology. They are "self-medicating" on what they need when they need it. And anyone who has a dog knows that they tend to eat grass when they have an upset stomach. Did they learn this at dog kindergarten? No, they just inherently know that it's what they need. I'm sure there was a time long ago when us humans were equally in tune with our biological needs. And actually, some humans still are: One of the last remaining hunter-gatherer people, the Hadza, will always eat the heart and the liver (the most nutritious parts) of the animal first. Right there on the spot after field dressing the animal. Oh and by the way, since this book is about body composition: yes, the Hadza are freakin shredded.

Maybe these biological cues can also explain some of the very weird cravings people sometimes get. Eating chalk as a kid is quite common, as is licking metal surfaces. Maybe, and this is me just speculating for fun, those kids are calcium and/or iron deficient?

EATING AND NOT EATING

Notice that diet and gut health are not the same thing. Diet contributes to good gut health but so do many other things. Gut health stands for your ability to take in nutrients, absorb those nutrients and expel whatever your body doesn't need. So it's a mixture of eating, not eating, ingesting and pooping. Hippocrates famously said "all disease begins in the gut" and this piece of ancient wisdom is being validated more and more every day. The gut microbiome, the bacteria living inside of you, is constantly being linked to various disease and health states with new studies coming out every day.

What you eat definitely matters a great deal when it comes to health, but more and more studies are pointing to the fact that abstaining from food at times might be even more important. Your body does different things when you're eating (or digesting) and when you're not eating, also called fasting. We all fast. Some people only fast for the time they're sleeping, some people also skip meals either intentionally or unintentionally. So it's good to understand that regardless of your lifestyle, you're already fasting sometimes. So what happens when you eat or don't eat? When you eat, the bulk of your body's energy at any given second is directed towards breaking that food down into usable pieces for the chemistry of life inside of you. Your body can't do anything with a piece of broccoli but it knows exactly what to do with all the phytonutrients, amino acids and other organic compounds that make up that piece of broccoli.

When you're fasting your body is not digesting food, so it can use all that extra energy towards something else. It starts to repair and recycle things. Every cell in your body has a lifespan and every single organ or system within the body needs to renew itself every so often. How do you renew something? You have to first break down the old stuff before you can build the new stuff. Fasting is a signal to the body that it's time to break some of this old stuff down. Conversely, eating is a signal that it's time to build new stuff to replace what was torn down. It's an elegant cycle of renewal that exists in every organism.

A lot of interesting research has been done on the benefits of fasting, and most of it is really recent. Dr Valter Longo has proven in mice and human studies that cycles of "fasting mimicking diet" can greatly improve markers of health and in mice even dramatically improve or dare I say cure "incurable" conditions such as multiple sclerosis or diabetes. Fasting mimicking diet is essentially a 5-day cycle of very low calories and as the name implies, the idea is to mimic "full" fasting but still allow the patients (or mice) to eat something.

Because fasting is an essential part of life in every organism, you should be mindful of it too. This doesn't necessarily mean that you need to devote extended periods of time to fasting, although that can be highly beneficial. Just think about the concept of eating and not eating and make sure your day includes plenty of both. For example: If you eat dinner at 9pm and then eat breakfast (the name of this meal comes from breaking your fast) at 7am you just did a 10-hour fast in between. If you ate dinner at 7pm and breakfast at 7am, you get a 12-hour fast. A good rule of thumb to aim for is that you should be fasting at least 12h every day. Which means you'll be eating during the other 12. Just keep in mind that any calories will break the fast. So if you put milk into your coffee in the morning, you are breaking your fast. If you drink that coffee black, it will have no calories and you're still in a fasted state afterwards. This 12/12 system is fairly easy to follow and it's beneficial to your body in a lot of ways which we'll get into later in this book. And as you remember from the sleep chapter, eating just before bed isn't a good idea anyway.

Extended fasting, basically anything more than 24 hours, is being heavily studied at the moment. The reason is clear: Fasting produces results that simply seem too good to be true. Stem cell activation, reversing autoimmune diseases, killing cancer cells and the list goes on and on. It's good to keep in mind that most of the research is being done on mice but there are quite a few human studies as well and the list keeps growing. In my opinion, fasting is one of the most powerful health promoting tools anyone has at their disposal but obviously more research is needed before general recommendations can really be made. There are some interesting hormone related studies though, more of those later in the chapters regarding weight loss and muscle building.

Study links:

https://www.ncbi.nlm.nih.gov/pubmed/?term=gut+micro-biome

https://www.ncbi.nlm.nih.gov/pubmed/?term=fasting+health

https://www.ncbi.nlm.nih.gov/pmc/articles/PMC4899145/

https://www.ncbi.nlm.nih.gov/pmc/?term=fasting+health

FOOD IS FUEL

So now let's actually talk about eating. Ingesting different foods always leads to different consequences within the body. For example, eating something with lots of protein (meat, eggs, tofu, etc) will lead to a spike in hormones and other messengers inside the body signaling growth. It's saying: We're getting lots of building blocks in, let's use them to build something. Insulin-like growth factor, IGF-1 and to a lesser extent insulin go up.

Eating something high in carbs (bread, potatoes, rice, etc) sends another signal: We're getting all this energy, let's fill up our energy stores. Or if those stores are already full, let's try to store up this energy. And the way your body stores energy is by creating more body fat. Even a fairly muscular big man can only store a few hundred grams of glucose (carbohydrates) into his muscles at any given time. Everything on top of that will be stored as body fat. The main signaling hormone responsible for storing energy in the body is insulin.

Eating foods high in fat (bacon, avocado, oils, etc) is similar to carbs in a sense that you're again giving your body a big shipment of energy. But there's a big difference: if you eat the fats with very little or no carbs at the same time, your body doesn't release much insulin. Without insulin it can't as efficiently store the fat you eat as body fat. It has to figure out other ways to use it. Or wait for other opportunities, such as another protein- or carb rich meal. People who usually eat diets higher in fat and lower in carbs can become quite good at burning fat as fuel inside their bodies. The same muscles that usually burn glucose as their main energy choice become good at burning fat as their energy of choice.

The main takeaway with proteins, carbs and fats is that it's important to understand their differences and what they are "meant to do". If carbs are mainly understood by your body to be energy, does it make sense to fuel up your body if you're not going to use this energy? Or in practical terms: If you're going to be sitting in the office all day, do you need to carb-up before that? Probably not. But if you're about to work out for an hour, having more carbs in your system might make a lot more sense. Same with protein: If you're eating all this protein, telling your body to grow, but you're not doing anything physical to send that muscle growth signal, your body doesn't really know what to do. And not all growth is good. For example cancer is an example of growth signals inside the body gone horribly wrong. That doesn't mean that protein causes cancer but tumors definitely use the same fuel sources as the rest of your body. There is a lot of exciting research happening now, investigating the link between the foods we eat and the cancers we diagnose and if we can in fact "starve out" cancer by not giving it what it wants.

So lifestyle to some extent should dictate what you eat. The more active you are, the more carbs you can "get away with", and the more protein you'll need. Fat is interesting because fats can be used in a variety of ways. If you're very used to eating lots of carbs and not much fat, you can get by with a fairly small fat intake. But some people, including me, operate better when they are limiting their carbohydrate intake but taking in lots of fat. The extreme version of this fat-centric approach is the ketogenic diet. Your body enters into a state of ketosis, converting fats into an energy source called 'ketone bodies', when you're basically eliminating all carbohydrates and only eating fats and protein. In this book I'm not getting into details regarding ketosis, a simple Google search will provide tons of info on the hows and whys behind it. Personally I feel better when I'm sliding in and out of ketosis (based on what my exercise routine looks like) and I always keep the carbs fairly low even if I'm not in ketosis.

So how can you figure out what makes sense for you? Well, are you trying to get smaller or bigger? If smaller, you probably don't want to be growth-signaling all the time. So keep the carbs low and protein intake moderate. Eat more fat to make up for the lost calories but keep the overall calories on the lower side. If you're trying to get bigger, it probably makes sense to increase the carbs and protein and bump up the calories. More on these strategies later in the book.

Your ancestry can also influence your ideal food choices: I'm from Finland, way high up North. My ancestors would've gone 6-9 months out of the year with very minimal carb intake simply because it's the winter time and there just are no plants available. Someone who's from Costa Rica would've been eating bananas all year long. It makes sense that Costa Ricans would be genetically better suited to eating the carbs in the bananas than Finns. Of course there are exceptions but as a general rule, this can be a good starting point to figuring out how you should fuel your body.

Study link:

https://www.ncbi.nlm.nih.gov/pmc/?term=fasting+cancer

FOOD IS NUTRITION

Of course the food you eat is not only fuel for the body, it's also the raw material are bodies are made of. Every cell in your body is made from the nutrients you eat. If your body is a factory, as we discussed before, you probably want to use high quality parts and raw materials to build that factory. So the first rule is to eat foods that are high in nutrition. By nutrition I mean vitamins, minerals and all the other millions of chemical compounds that exist in plants and animals. The more processed the food is, the less nutrients it's going to have. Processing includes things like slicing, grinding, drying, frying, heating, freezing, and so on. A potato picked from the ground has a lot of nutrients. A cut, deep-fried, frozen and then re-fried french fry is going to have less. Note that this same logic applies to cooking oils. Cold-pressed olive oil is just that: squeezed olives. Canola oil has gone through several steps of processing before it's bottled in the neutral tasting liquid form you're buying it from the grocery store. Processing will always reduce the nutritional value of a given food and can even turn it harmful.

So you'll want to favor foods that are minimally processed. This means mainly shopping in the vegetable and meat isles of the grocery store and skipping all the rest. If you're vegetarian or vegan, put more focus on the vegetable section of course. Only use olive oil, avocado oil, butter, ghee, coconut oil and other natural oils in cooking. Skip canola and soybean oil and other heavily processed fats. Another way to think about this is that you'll want to avoid "empty calories", meaning foods that are high in calories but low in nutrients. An avocado has a lot of calories but it also has a lot of nutrition so it's a good choice. Almonds are heavy in calories but have a lot of nutrients, again a good choice. A bag of potato chips has a lot of calories but minimal nutrients so it's a bad choice. A bag of candy is even worse. You get the idea.

There's a certain amount of commonly recognised vitamins and minerals that pretty much everyone agrees we need to obtain on a regular basis. You'll probably know most of these: It's vitamins like vitamin A, B-vitamins, vitamin C and so on. Minerals like magnesium, calcium, potassium, etc. What you probably didn't know is that almost nobody gets even the recommended official minimum daily amount of all these vitamins and minerals from the foods they eat. Vitamins and minerals are commonly added to foods like breakfast cereals, milk and so on to boost these levels in people on a population level. But most people still end up with deficiencies somewhere. The reasons actually aren't 100% clear but it looks like just eating a vitamin or mineral in some form doesn't guarantee that you're actually getting that stuff into your body in a usable form. For example if you take a vitamin B2 supplement, your pee will turn yellow. That's because you're peeing most of that vitamin B2 out. Maybe all of it. Simply adding vitamins and minerals into food as supplements, or taking supplements doesn't guarantee that your body knows what to do with those nutrients.

Now when you obtain those nutrients from natural foods, they're never alone, isolated and hyper condensed like with supplements. Fat-soluble vitamins in nature are always found together with fats, which makes sense because that's how your body can take those vitamins in. If you just eat fat-soluble vitamins without fat, they go to waste. Fat-soluble vitamins include vitamin A and D. In nature you'll find both of those vitamins in pretty good levels in for example fish liver, which again is also fatty. There's also a huge list of other nutrients, besides the commonly recognised vitamins and minerals, that exist in plants and animals. A lot of newer research is pointing to the fact that this nutrient puzzle is a lot more complex than is commonly appreciated. Nutrients behave differently in the absence of other ones and vice versa. Example: Studies show that curcumin will increase glutathione, your body's master antioxidant and this elevated glutathione will make your body's vitamin C cycling more efficient which means you'll need less vitamin C to get the same result as before. So if you eat curcumin, your vitamin C minimum requirement theoretically goes down. Or let's look at calcium: Everyone "knows" that calcium is important to your bones, right? But did you know that calcium by itself doesn't really do anything to your bones. You need correct amounts of other nutrients like vitamin D and K2 to actually ensure that the calcium you eat goes where it should.

Now all of that is a very complicated way to get back to the same message as before: You should eat real foods high in nutrients. It's your best bet to try and get everything you need and simply by eating this way you're already way ahead of the curve.

I've personally gone through quite rigorous nutrient lab testing because I really wanted to turn every stone and see where I'm at. After running an organic acids panel (urine and blood tests) I discovered I had an elevated need of vitamins B2, B3 and C and minerals magnesium, manganese and zinc and few other chemical compounds like alpha-lipoic acid and glutathione. At the time I was eating tons of plants and high quality meat and I was still deficient in quite a few things. This brings us to the next topic: your ability to actually absorb nutrients.

Study link:

https://www.ncbi.nlm.nih.gov/pubmed/15650394

ABSORBING FOOD

Even after you chew and swallow food, the food is still actually outside your body. Your stomach is essentially a tube that goes from mouth to anus. The only way for the food to actually get into your body is through the permeable gut lining. It is an elegant and genius barrier that filters everything you eat. Things your body recognises as nutrients get passed through and other stuff gets blocked and pooped out. Or rather, this is how it should work. But clearly in modern times this system goes haywire often. Just look at the number of food intolerances, allergies and autoimmune diseases which are all rising heavily in the developed countries. What all those three things have in common is that they are all triggered by particles that the body views as threats and attacks them. But really, particles like that shouldn't get into your body in the first place if the gut barrier was working correctly.

Time to revisit my own personal story a bit: I damaged my gut and problems in that realm eventually launched me on my health freak journey. In 2012 I went on a trip to Indonesia with my friends and had a great time except for one little thing: I got a salmonella infection. I got a high fever, couldn't keep any food in, the usual fun stuff. I got some antibiotics from a local pharmacy and the immediate symptoms cleared enough for me to travel back home. Back in Finland I got a medical lab test done which confirmed the salmonella and I took more antibiotics. I got better in a couple of weeks and went back to my old ways which included quite a bid of foods that I now wouldn't touch with a stick: pizza, ice cream, candy, deep-fried garbage and of course alcohol every weekend. After about a month, I got quite sick again so I went to the doctor's. Figured the salmonella wasn't completely gone. But no, the test came back negative. Doctor couldn't really figure out what was going on and just told me to wait it out. And I waited for months. My stomach was a complete mess all the time, I lost weight and just felt like crap all the time. Doctors had no answers, they even tested me for celiac disease but that also came back negative. After awhile I couldn't take it anymore and was willing to try dramatic measures to get better. So for the first time in my life I went on a diet: a gluten-free diet. And boom, magically in a couple of days I started to feel better. A lot better. I was convinced. After awhile I found out about the paleo diet, where you eliminate "modern" foods like grains, dairy and pretty much anything processed, tried that and I started to feel even better. Obviously this was a big lifestyle change: I had to start cooking a lot more and eating out way less. Treats and snacks changed from candy and potato chips to an apple and kale chips.

I've now been eating a strict paleo diet for 8 years. And the reason I'm not even thinking about going back to my old ways is that not only did this lifestyle fix my gut problems, it also helped with unexpected things: I felt more energetic, slept better, my migraines decreased significantly and my skin basically never breaks out anymore. Clearly my gut barrier started to work again. And of course over time my body composition significantly changed: more muscle and less fat.

FOOD IS ALSO FEEDING YOUR GUT BACTERIA

So why was the paleo diet a magical cure for me all of a sudden? We'll never know for sure but I very much suspect it has to do with the next topic of discussion: The gut microbiome. Every human carries around about 2 kg or 4-5 pounds of bacteria with you all the time. Trillions of bacteria. These critters live on your skin, in your mouth and mostly in your gut. They live in a symbiotic relationship with you: You feed them, they feed you. You provide them with a home, they clean up that home. The whole topic of gut microbiome is still very poorly understood, mainly because only recently have we developed tools that are accurate enough to actually detect and study these little guys. One thing seems quite clear though: gut microbiome is very important and it wouldn't be unfair to even call it an organ. That's right, the gut microbiome can be compared in its importance to your liver, kidneys or even the heart or the brain.

When I took those antibiotics to wipe out the salmonella infection, I basically carpet bombed my gut microbiome, killing everything in sight. I got rid of the salmonella but also a lot of the good guys that are supposed to inhabit my gut. When I then went back to my old unhealthy habits, I started a negative chain reaction by putting in things that I had no ability to deal with anymore. The reason why I could eat all the gluten in the world previously without a problem was most likely the fact that I had millions of little helpers in my gut. I was probably always as bad at digesting gluten as I am now, but my gut bacteria took care of it. I wasn't eating it, but they were. Same with sugar, dairy and even alcohol. Another very plausible explanation is that the gut bacteria actually are a functional part of your gut lining. Maybe the gut bacteria had been working overtime all my life, fixing things that I was breaking with my lifestyle. Your body has essentially outsourced some tasks to the gut bacteria. If the gut bacteria are not there anymore to send signals back to your body, the whole system starts to malfunction. There is a lot of interesting ongoing research in this field of back and forth communication between your body and the bacteria inside it.

What we now know from endless studies is that pretty much everything you do changes your gut bacteria. That's obvious when it comes to things like your diet but also applies to lifestyle. If you go out for a run, your gut bacteria will change. If you get depressed, your gut bacteria change. If you get a good night's sleep, your gut bacteria will change. Remember the analogy of your body as a factory? It now seems pretty clear that your gut bacteria are also machinery in that factory. They synthesise nutrients and actively take part in your metabolism, providing you with things your body needs and taking care of stuff that's left over. As if human metabolism wasn't complex enough, we now understand that human metabolism is actually a collaboration between the human and trillions of other life forms. In fact, there's way more bacterial DNA inside you than human DNA, and to complicate things even further, we now know that the bacteria can also swap DNA back and forth with you.

And I wiped most of that metabolic machinery out with the super aggressive antibiotic regime I took. Now since then I've had my gut microbiome tested a few times to see what creatures actually reside inside of me. There are quite a few companies that provide this service, I've mainly used uBiome. It has been very interesting and encouraging to see that the gut microbiome indeed does change dramatically over time. Even though I'm not eating gluten anymore, I've still managed to even get a pretty decent population of gluten-consuming bacteria back in there. Most likely these same bacteria can survive on other things beside the gluten as well, because clearly something in my diet is feeding them.

So I think we can now agree that gut microbiome is very important and you should also think about feeding the bacteria with your diet. So how do you do that? Again, a pretty commonly known "fact" is that fiber is good for your gut and that it feeds the gut microbiome. This is sort of true. There are lots of bacterial species that we 100% know feed on the fiber you eat from food. This is also pretty easy to validate for yourself: Eat lots of garlic or beans, both high in types of fiber the bacteria like and you'll soon discover that you're gassy. Like really gassy. This is because the bacteria will consume that fiber, thrive in this abundant environment, rapidly multiply, and poop out gas like crazy. Which all builds up in your stomach and needs to get out somehow. But fiber is not the whole story when it comes to improving your gut microbiome. We just discussed that bacteria also change with lifestyle changes. Some bacterial species might even increase when you go on a fast and eat nothing for a few days. The interactions between your body and the gut microbiome are so complex that anyone who claims to fully understand it is just flat out lying. We still have no idea about everything going on.

It only makes sense that the best way to look after your microbial buddies is to look after their home "planet", you. The best diet for your gut microbiome is what's best for you. You shouldn't try to eat in a way that's "scientifically proven to be the for the best gut microbiome" if it makes you feel like crap. If you don't feel good, you'll just grow and harbor a bacterial population that is very good at making you feel bad. When I personally changed my diet and started to "create more health" inside of me, I also started to foster and grow a new bacterial population that has that same goal in mind. That's why my gut bacteria looks different in the lab tests I took: it's the perfect one for me right now.

Study link:

https://www.ncbi.nlm.nih.gov/pubmed/?term=gut+micro-biome+changes

Summary

- Respect your ancestry when it comes to food choices
- There's more to food than just taste
- Regularly fast for at least 10 hours every day (night)
- Fuel your body based on it's needs
- Eat mainly whole real nutrient-dense foods
- Take care of your gut microbiome by taking care of your body

CHAPTER 2.3 STRESS

ADDICTED TO STRESS

Stress kills. Stress is the new smoking. I'm sure you've heard something along those lines before. And it makes sense: Being stressed isn't fun, right? No, actually there are tons of people that are addicted to stress. Being stressed can actually feel great! You get a rush in adrenaline and cortisol, powerful substances that make you feel alive and in the moment. You feel energetic, you can run through obstacles, crush at work, go full beast mode in the gym. Until you do this long enough and one day you just can't anymore, and then you sit there and wonder what happened.

We're an overstressed society but it's not only because of external pressures. We do it to ourselves all the time. We drink tons of coffee, we work too much, we compensate for working too much by working out too much, we party all the time and we go on adventures on our holidays. We're trying to achieve all the time. But all stress is stress. There is no "positive stress" and "negative stress". There's just stress. When you're asking your body to work hard, it is stressful. And by the way, thinking hard is just as demanding for the body as exercising hard. There are even anecdotes that show a hugely increased calorie expenditure for professional chess players, just from all that thinking and sitting still. In my personal opinion one of the craziest misconceptions about health is that your body and mind are somehow different entities. What's good for your physical conditioning is good for your brain. You can't meditate your way to good brain health if all you do is sit on a pillow every day. This is again one of those things that is only fairly recently being proven in studies. Exercising before a cognitive test improves working memory, going for a walk in nature makes you smarter, and so on.

Why are we talking about brain health when the topic is stress? Because your brain's ability to handle stress is very much tied to your physical conditioning. When you're active, using your muscles, pumping blood through the system you are "mobilizing" those stress hormones. They are doing what they're supposed to be doing. Your body has the ability to get stressed because it's a life saving ability. When an animal notices a threat, their heart rate elevates, their senses sharpen and their stress hormones spike: They're ready to fight to the death, or run away. They're tapping into their sympathetic nervous system. As opposed to the parasympathetic "rest and digest" system where they normally operate in.

When you drink a cup of coffee and walk into a work meeting to discuss a problem, your body gets ready to fight, or flee. You're a bit anxious and combative but also efficient and strong. So you feel good, you'll get your point across, maybe overpower the other person with your arguments and walk out of the meeting room as a "winner". And you just stressed the hell out of your body that was working hard for that whole hour, getting ready for any possible outcome, including physical violence. After the high from the meeting starts to wear off, you'll start to feel a bit tired so you grab another cup of coffee before the next meeting and here we go again.

In the animal kingdom, stress lasts for a few seconds and then it's gone. In the human domain, stress seems to last for 70 years and then you die. Animals also unconsciously, or maybe even consciously, do things to alleviate stress: When a dog is stressed about something for a bit, it'll shake its whole body for a couple of seconds and magically it's happy again, wagging its tail. The dog is mobilizing the cortisol and giving its nervous system a nice shake to relax the muscles. The body gets these cues and calms down. We modern humans rarely actively engage in anti-stress activities through our day, we just go from one stressful activity to the next without a pause in between. Our ancestors were a lot smarter. That's why some cultures still practice "siestas" for example where, usually from noon to 1pm, where everything shuts down and people just take an hour to relax.

Study links:

https://www.menshealth.com/fitness/a29144951/chess-players-calorie-burn/

https://www.ncbi.nlm.nih.gov/pmc/articles/PMC5934999/

THE AUTONOMIC NERVOUS SYSTEM

Your autonomic nervous system controls autonomous (automatic) behaviours in the body, such as breathing. You don't think about breathing, you just breathe. That autonomic nervous system has two "modes": sympathetic and parasympathetic. As we discussed in the previous chapter, the sympathetic nervous system is the "fight or flight" mode, meant to only really be tapped into when it's a matter of life and death. Most of the time, any organism would be in the parasympathetic "rest and digest" mode, chilling out and digesting food. It's not quite as black and white as it sounds, but any activity will mainly fall under one of these umbrellas. And sometimes the same activity can be both: Let's take something like snowboarding down a hill as an example. If you're just cruising, enjoying the sun and the scenery and laughing with friends, this will be seen by the body mainly as a parasympathetic restful activity, even if you're still using your muscles and elevating your heart rate. If you're bombing down the hill hard and fast, struggling to see what's ahead of you because of the heavy snowfall, your body is hard on the sympathetic side of things, fighting to keep you alive.

Because the autonomic nervous system controls involuntary things like breathing and heartbeat, measuring these things can tell you if your body is in a relaxed state or not. Again, there is some cool new technology which can help quite a bit. Measuring something called HRV, heart rate variability, can give you quite a straightforward answer to how stressed you are. In a relaxed state your heart is supposed to beat in unsteady intervals. A metronome-like steady beat is a sign of sympathetic activation, ie stress. The tricky thing with measuring HRV is that it's something that should be done first thing in the morning before anything stressful has happened to you. Few years ago I tried measuring my HRV every morning by strapping a heart-rate monitor on my chest before I even got out of bed. It definitely worked and was valuable info but after a month or so I stopped doing it. Just too much hassle. But thankfully the Oura ring we discussed in the sleep chapter also measures HRV. And it does it automatically, every night. As do many other wearable trackers. This is what the HRV measurement from Oura ring looks like:

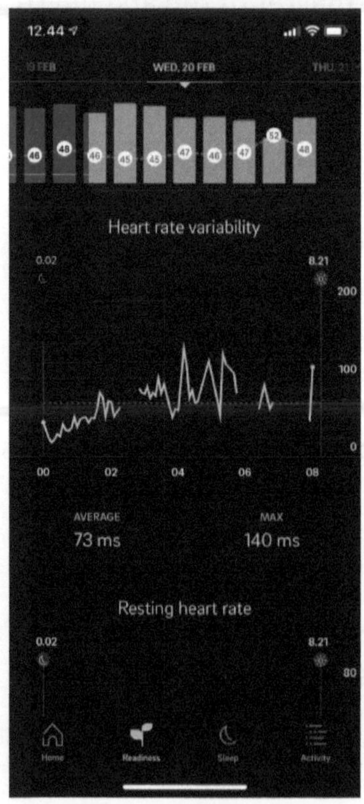

The exact numbers you should aim for are basically irrelevant because they vary heavily from person to person. But on a personal level they are very valuable. For me, that was a great night, which means that nothing was stressing me on a chronic level. I can clearly see my HRV numbers steadily dropping if I exercise more than usual, work more than usual or have some sort of personal problems going on. Similarly, taking it easy for a bit by going on a holiday will lead to a rise in HRV. The higher the HRV, generally the less stressed your body is. Technology isn't magically going to fix anything but I do find it to be very helpful in identifying problems before they arise. Tracking things like HRV and sleep allows me to see where I'm trending and I can change my behaviour accordingly before anything really goes wrong. Poor night of sleep and low HRV? Okay, today is not the day to go after that personal record deadlift. I might still go to the gym but I'll focus on less taxing exercises. Great night's sleep and skyhigh HRV? This is a great day to take on more stressful activities.

You should think about your life, routines and what you do and try to map out everything on this spectrum. How many parasympathetic and sympathetic activities can you count on a daily or a weekly basis and is it heavily skewed in either direction? Some people will naturally gravitate towards a lot of sympathetic things, other people will be pretty relaxed by nature and tend to stick to things that are calm and quiet. Personally I need to make a conscious effort to include more parasympathetic things in my life. I'm what you could call a "cortisol junkie". I'm addicted to those chemicals and hormones that make me feel alive and like I'm always doing something. I struggle with just relaxing and letting things just happen. Usually people like me also tend to suffer from things like insomnia because it's harder for us to just relax. But we have no problem getting motivated to go to the gym. Anything to keep the boredom away. Think about where you fall on this spectrum and try to balance your activities out to include a healthy balance of sympathetic and parasympathetic activity.

Meditation is often touted as a great way to relax and balance out your mind. The studies on meditation and its benefits are overwhelmingly positive, no question about it. It's the bomb and everyone should try it at least. Personally I've read books about the subject, tried various structured meditation programs and even had a streak where I meditated every day for 7 months straight. I went as far as to buy a device called Muse that measures your brain waves during meditation. And even after 7 months it felt I wasn't getting any better at it. Meditation is definitely the hardest health practice I've ever encountered. I find it easier to go without food for 5 days than to sit still with my thoughts for 20 minutes. Even writing that feels kind of crazy and just underlines the point that I need to meditate more. My personal meditation journey is still just beginning. Bodybuilder Ben Pakulski has a great motto which I've incorporated into my life: 'If I can't, I must'. The things that are the hardest will benefit you the most.

Regardless of whether you meditate in a structured manner, there's great value in "programming" relaxing parasympathetic activities into your life consciously. These activities can be anything, but they can't be two things. Let me explain. Multitasking is the enemy of being mindful. Even something as simple as taking a walk and listening to a podcast is not as relaxing as just taking a walk. Your attention will be split and you're not fully listening to the podcast or enjoying the scenery. One thing at a time. Even doing the dishes can be relaxing and peaceful if you're mindfully just experiencing the feeling of water, the motion of rubbing the plates clean and the reward of the accomplishment. Personally I like to take walks in the forest, with or without my dog. Sometimes I just lay down on the couch listening to music. Simply being there with nothing to achieve, just enjoying the experience. Find what works for you.

Study link:

https://www.ncbi.nlm.nih.gov/pmc/?term=meditation

STAYING SOCIAL

The human animal is a social animal. The most severe form of punishment in our society is extreme isolation. The worst criminals get thrown into a jail cell without access to any other humans for most of the day. And as a result those guys often go crazy. Or crazier I should say.

It seems pretty obvious that social contact therefore is crucial for proper hormone function as well. And indeed it is. Nothing lowers your cortisol like laughing with friends. Or even seeing a smiling face. We have something called "mirror neurons" inside us which do exactly what the name suggests: They mirror what they see. When you watch someone surfing, some part of your brain is experiencing what they are experiencing. You'll feel some part of that thrill. When you see someone smiling at you, you'll inherently want to smile back. Remember that hormones are feelings and all feelings evoke a hormonal response. You become happier as a result.

Then there are the obvious examples: Having sex raises testosterone in both men and women. And conversely having high testosterone creates a higher sex drive. Even seeing a beautiful woman (or a man) will raise testosterone. As a man you might then assume that it's good to hang out with beautiful women if you want to have high testosterone. And it probably would be a good strategy. But testosterone will also go up in prison with nothing but other dudes around. On studies done with straight men I might add. So what's up with that? Well one of the biggest elevators of testosterone is competition, especially with other men. This might help explain why testosterone generally drops in married men, compared to single men. Less competition and less need for high testosterone levels.

Please don't get divorced to elevate your testosterone. But maybe you could use some more male comradery and competition in your life? Next time you're going to the gym, grab a buddy with you. Social contact will help push you a bit further with your workout and laughing about it afterwards will help bring that cortisol down.

Study links

https://www.sciencedirect.com/science/article/abs/pii/019188699400177T

Summary

- Stress often feels good and that's what it makes it so addictive
- Don't pour more stress on stress. All stress is stress
- Measuring things like HRV can be very valuable tools in managing stress
- Identify parasympathetic and sympathetic activities in your life and strive for balance
- Stay social

CHAPTER 2.4
MOVEMENT

YOUR BRAIN MOVES YOU

One fundamental truth about all movement: It always originates in the brain. Your mind and your body are interlinked in every way possible. Without the mind, muscles are useless. In fact, brain development in an infant happens mainly through movement. After all, moving towards or away from something is the first step in learning anything. Because your brain is shaped by your body movement, moving your body is one of the best ways to take care of your brain. You might know that Parkinson's disease symptoms are caused by lack of dopamine due to death of so called "dopaminergic neurons". No dopamine, no movement. Conversely in a healthy person, movement will trigger dopamine. Or rather dopamine spikes just before the movement is initiated. The thought to move, conscious or unconscious, spikes dopamine and initiates the movement.

Most movement problems therefore are neurological, at least in part. This might sound bad but it's actually good news. It means that if you fixed your back pain, you actually fixed your brain. Who wouldn't want a healthier brain?

AVOIDING ACHES
AND PAINS

Your body is an adaptation machine. Any time you do anything, including sitting down reading this book right now, your body is getting better at it. You're becoming a better book reading machine. Now, chances are a book reading machine isn't going to look all that hot, so maybe get up and stretch your legs a bit.

Kidding aside, the biggest thing regarding movement practice and health really is that: movement. What happens for most of the day is what matters most. You can't exercise your way to good physical health if all you do for the rest of the day is lying down. As with sleep, technology can be our worst enemy but also our ally: Almost any phone will have a built-in step counter nowadays and there are a gazillion different smartwatches and activity trackers on the market. You can't fix a problem if you don't know one exists, so getting a baseline read on your activity level is very helpful. So get a device and test it out. If you're regularly getting 10 000 or more steps throughout the day, you're doing ok. 10 000 isn't a magical number by any means and you shouldn't stop there, but it's an easy-to-remember nice round number to aim at. If you're falling below 10 000 consistently, take actions to move more. Drive less, move more, go for walks. Park your car further away. Leave the train earlier and walk the rest of the way. It's not rocket science.

Walking is a fundamental human movement so it makes sense to measure daily steps but the same principle of movement applies to the rest of your body. If you are the average person, chances are quite high that you suffer from tight shoulders and neck and probably some back pain as well. The reason isn't because you suffer from a chiropractic deficiency or because you have bad back genes, it's because you're not using the muscles that control your shoulders, neck, hips, legs and back enough so you end up with unbalanced muscles. Unbalanced muscles create unstable environments and the body tries to create stability by creating tension. And now your lower back hurts. Or you can't turn your head.

Now, it's good to understand one very fundamental principle when it comes to tight muscles: All muscle tightness is neurological in origin. That means that (unless you had physical injury torn muscle) there is nothing physically "stuck" or "wrong" in the muscle itself. The nerves that control the muscle are constantly sending that muscle a signal that says "contract" and the muscle follows orders. This is why getting a massage feels good in the moment but usually only for a little bit and then you're feeling tight again. By applying pressure and touch to the muscle, the masseuse was able to make the nerves relax and the muscle relaxed as a consequence. But since they did nothing to affect the root cause of the issue, it comes right back. And the root cause usually lies in a muscle imbalance somewhere in the system. If you don't believe me, look for Annette Verpillot's TedX talk mentioned in the Resources and Recommendations (chapter 5) and perform the eye tracking exercise right now. If you got any pain and tightness, chances are you will be blown away by the results.

As with all the other chapters, the focus here is on the big rocks. We're not going to get into the details of how to fix every possible muscle tightness problem but rather let's focus on easy things that will help most people the most. The best way to avoid muscle imbalances is to move in a balanced way and do that often. When you're reading this book, you're going to be hunched over forwards for some time. Your neck will get tighter, your shoulders and pecs will twist forward and your biceps will be activated. To balance this out, you should also do something that counters these forces. Straighten your back, look up, spread your arms wide, move them back and forth, bring your shoulders down. When you're at work, try not to stay in one position all day. Stand up sometimes, sit down on an office chair other times and maybe just lounge for a bit. In between, take a walk.

Of course the most powerful way to address muscle imbalances is to physically train the muscles. Strength training, when done correctly, is a fantastic way to maintain good posture and overall balanced physique. But if done incorrectly, it can be a very powerful way to mess yourself up even more. People often gravitate towards the kind of exercise they're naturally good at. In a gym environment this is very obvious. Usually when people start going to the gym, they try out all kinds of different exercises. Soon they discover that they like this and that exercise but dislike some other ones. So they tend to stick with the movements they like and ignore the rest. Over time this will simply make your imbalances even worse because you are strengthening those existing patterns inside your body and weakening the counteracting forces. A practical example: Let's say you love the bench press and building your chest but don't like things like cable or barbell rows which would target your upper back. So you tend to neglect the back exercises but never skip chest day. After awhile you will develop overactive shoulders and chest that will start to roll your posture forward. Meanwhile the muscles that are supposed to hold your shoulders down and back become weak and underactive. You will eventually develop an unbalanced posture and your risk of injury goes up over time. Balanced exercise programming is crucial.

Somewhat ironically the worst offenders in creating unbalanced and achy bodies tend to be hobbies, be it physical activities like soccer, ice hockey, tennis or non physical activities like playing computer games. The reason should be pretty obvious by now: Whenever you do something often, your body gets really good at that one specific thing. So for example a hockey player is going to be pretty good at leaning to the left or to the right all the time, twisting their body in one way with maximum strength and using their feet in a very specific way to skate really fast. Doesn't sound like a very balanced body. Usually even when athletic people "pull their back" or just generally hurt themselves by doing something very mundane, the warning signs were all there well before the injury happened. We just don't tend to think about the benefits of not being injured, until we actually are injured. But as with everything, it's way easier to avoid a problem in the body than to fix it later. Taking care of your meat machine is always a good investment.

TO CARDIO OR NOT TO CARDIO

Everyone's heard of cardio, shorthand for cardiovascular exercise, usually meaning running or biking for a long time with a pretty steady speed. It's hailed as the one magical way to train your most important muscle: the heart. Also it burns tons of calories which means you'll be burning fat like crazy. Both of those things are simply wrong. If someone likes running or biking, there is nothing wrong with that and everyone should be free to do whatever makes them feel good, but it's very dangerous to preach the wonders of cardio as the magic fix for everything for everyone.

How many people do you know who's only exercise modality is going running? Chances are you know quite a lot of people like that. How many of those people are in great physical shape? Chances are, not that many. There are a number of problems with "chronic cardio" where cardiovascular activity is one's only true exercise modality. Let's start with an obvious one. We just discussed how your body adapts to whatever you're doing most often. Running or biking are very leg-dominant exercises so you're pretty much neglecting the rest of your body. But even worse is the fact that most people simply don't know how to run well. Almost nobody thinks of running as a skill that you should practice. We just go for a run. But most people will have muscle imbalances that will affect their running gait and even 30 minutes of running consists of thousands of repetitions. Tens of thousands of faulty repetitions of one legged jumps (which is what running essentially is) every week is a recipe for disaster. That's why there are terms like "runner's knee", which is just a knee injury. This is also why every sports sneaker store will have specialists who can diagnose some problem with your running gait and then "fix it" by selling you a sneaker which addresses the fact that your feet pronate or supinate. You'll buy the new shoe and for awhile it feels great to run again before another part of your body breaks down. The shoe didn't fix anything. It just directed the energy of your faulty gait somewhere else.

"But wait Joonas, aren't you this paleo guy and aren't humans made for running", you say. And you are correct. Humans are excellent at running long distances. We can outrun almost any animal. If, and this is a huge if, we have been doing that all our life. Almost nobody in the modern western environment has been a runner ever since they were a little kid and even those people were wearing shoes from when they learned to walk. We modern humans just don't have the feet that "original humans" did. The human foot is an excellent design: it's got great shock absorbers, it can grip things and the skin is unbelievably resistant to almost anything. But the foot of a modern human is soft, weak and dysfunctional. Here's an easy analogy: How do you think your hands would work and look like if you had been wearing mittens your whole life? Or even more accurately: a cast. The modern shoes most people wear are very rigid and stable, so the foot just atrophies. There's no reason for the foot to maintain a strong arch, powerful and nimble toes or a hard damage-resistant skin. Our bodies adapt to what we do, and our feet have adapted to doing pretty much nothing. Not to worry though, feet can be trained like every other part of the body. But you need to take it slow. Start by walking more barefoot, get flatter shoes and over time work towards exercising barefoot or in minimalist shoes. This will prevent a lot of problems down the line.

Another problem with this chronic cardio is that it doesn't really work all that well for creating a better body, internally or externally. Let's start with the internal side of things. The general misunderstanding is that cardiovascular exercise targets your heart better than any other form of exercise and it's important to do cardio to have a healthy heart. Again, this is simply wrong. Any exercise or activity that elevates your heart rate will "target" your heart as well as cardio does. But all forms of exercise do something else besides elevating your heart rate: They will force your body to adapt. The adaptation you get from cardio is being able to go a little bit further or a little bit faster next time. It's a very slow gradual signal to the body. If instead of cardio you did for example high intensity interval training, or HIIT for short, you would send a signal to the body that it will need to change significantly to be able to handle a much greater workload that it's used to. HIIT consists of short bursts of all-out full speed sprints followed by a long rest period. A HIIT workout might look like this for example: after warming up run full speed for 30 seconds, jog or walk very slowly for 3 minutes, run full speed for 30 seconds, jog very slowly for 3 minutes, run full speed for 30 seconds, and jog home slowly. A HIIT workout will take 10 to 15 minutes and will actually do more for your VO2Max (your maximum oxygen intake capability) than pretty much any amount of cardiovascular training. It will also build strength, speed up your metabolism and burn fat in the process. And what about the heart? Well in the HIIT workout the heart is literally working to its full capacity for a short time, then recovering for a long time so it can do that again. It's literally the same exercise modality as strength training, and since the heart is a muscle like any other muscle, it will grow stronger with this way of training.

What about external qualities? Cardio training alone doesn't make you sexy, sorry. The signal that it sends to the body is "we need to be able to do this monotonous activity for a long time".

It will adapt to make you look like a long distance runner. You won't need any upper body strength so forget about muscular or toned arms, chest, shoulders or back. Your legs need to be light and efficient so no need for a lot of muscle there either. But at least it'll make you skinny, right? Wrong. The one good thing about body fat is that it's a great fuel source for a long run. Humans don't accidentally store body fat in the places that are optimal for a bipedal organism: around the belly, butt and thighs. It's a genius system that will allow humans to store extra energy from their food and go for a long time without food when needed, because carrying fat around doesn't really hinder our performance. When you engage in chronic cardio you're sending a signal to the body that we'll have a high need for an extra fuel source so better keep that safety cushion around. It's quite common to see people on the treadmill or on a running trail that seem to be in great shape but also have quite a high body fat percentage. Most of them wonder why they struggle to lose this stubborn fat so they run or bike longer and harder. It's because their goal doesn't match with their exercise modality. If their goal is to run 10km, great job. If their goal is to lose weight, they are just literally spinning their wheels. More on exercise and fat loss in the following chapters.

There is of course also another side to this cardio story: When done properly it's a great health promoting tool. If you are a great and efficient runner with perfect technique, jogging 10km a few times a week is fantastic. It'll get the blood pumping, clearing out all kinds of gunk from your body, increasing cool stuff like Brain Derived Neurotrophic Factor (which is basically like Miracle Grow for the brain), it'll help you sleep better, improve your mood and decision making and so on. The list is long. BUT any kind of exercise will accomplish most of these things. So again the story with cardio really is that any exercise is beneficial and useful, not just the cardio type exercise. If you feel like going for a run, do it. I bet you'll feel great. But don't get duped by the "marketing". Running is just one form of exercise and too much of anything can turn a great thing bad.

EXERCISE MOTIVATION

The main reason why most people quit going to fitness classes or stop seeing their personal trainer is that they are not seeing results. They have goals in mind, realistic or not, and after awhile they just don't see the value in beating themselves up for nothing. And that's 100% understandable: Why would you do something you don't like if it's not even working? This conversation brings us back to the topic of adaptation. When most people work out, they are not really adapting. They are just causing damage, recovering and going back to cause more damage. The adaptations that are happening are so small that they don't cause any visible changes. I was also stuck in this hole for years. I went to the gym very regularly, did my workouts but nothing was really changing. I was already decently fit so it wasn't the end of the world. I still looked pretty good naked and was strongish for my size, so I just figured that I'm at the peak of my potential. I was definitely wrong. When I changed my exercise programming to something that is actually thought through and most importantly started tracking my workouts, I suddenly started to make a lot of progress. More on exercise programming in the weight loss and muscle building chapters, but let's talk about tracking your workouts. When I talk to people about fitness, I often hear that they don't know if their exercise routine is working. I find this kind of crazy. If you simply track your weights for a month, you'll 100% know if you are getting stronger or not. Getting stronger means your workout routine is working. Not getting stronger means it's not working.

I don't care what kind of exercise you do, lifting weights, running, swimming or yoga, if you're not tracking your progress in one way or another, you're missing out on a huge piece of the fitness puzzle: intrinsic motivation.

Relying on being externally motivated is a terrible way to get anything done. Imagine what your dental health would look like if you just relied on external motivation in brushing your teeth. "I'll just brush my teeth when I feel like it. Lately I've had a hard time picking that brush up". Everyone agrees that's a depressed or a crazy person. But we tend to accept this as a reality when it comes to exercise. What people miss is that you can also create more motivation. Your motivation to brushing your teeth probably comes from two things: you don't want to look or smell bad, and you want to keep your teeth healthy. The first one is probably a bigger reason why you brush your teeth, but it also feels good to know that it's healthy for you. The same exact paradigm could apply to exercising: You exercise because you want to look better and also it's nice that it's healthy. So why is it harder to get motivated to go to the gym than to brush your teeth? The gym is a bigger investment of time and effort, and the reward maybe isn't as obvious and quick as with brushing your teeth. But what if you could actually see those results right away like with brushing your teeth? Now the formula changes: You don't need to do something for an hour to get a better body eventually. You WANT to do something for an hour to get a better body eventually.

And this is where tracking your results comes in. It's the 100% guaranteed way to see results instantly when you exercise. And it's so simple: Simple write down what you're doing at the gym (or on the running trail) every time you do it. *I was lifting weights last week and when I lift weights today, I can see I'm stronger than I was a week ago.* Knowing that you're on the right path spikes your dopamine and cements this pattern to your brain: *I lift weights, I get a reward, I like lifting weights, I want to lift more weights to get more rewards*. After a while you also see changes in your body, which spikes dopamine further, strengthening this positive feedback loop. And next thing you know, you're now a super motivated legit gym rat, working out every day and actually probably need to cut down your training a bit. If this is you, revisit the stress chapter.

MINIMUM EFFECTIVE DOSE

On a general population level, people for sure don't exercise enough. But the flipside is that the people who exercise regularly, usually do too much of it. "Minimum effective dose to elicit the most amount of change" is a fascinating concept that I don't hear being used nearly enough. Simply put it means doing just the right amount of something and then stopping there. It's great advice for pretty much everything in life, but if it applies to anything, it applies to exercise. And it's really simple: Every time you work out, lift just enough weights to see your numbers go up from last time and stop there. Or run fast enough to see your 5k time drop and don't run any more. Leave some gas in the tank and come back even stronger or faster tomorrow. Recovery is crucial.

One of the better analogies for understanding the concept of minimum effective dose is tanning. If you want to get tanned are you better off A) going full beast mode and staying in the sun all day or B) slowly increasing your sun exposure over days? Obviously B. Option A will leave you burned and hurting, and will keep you out of the sun for the next few days while you're recovering from your stupidity.

WORKING OUT AND WORKING IN

Speaking of recovery, let's talk about the concept of working out and working in. We all know what working out refers to but what's this weird "working in"? Remember how in the stress chapter we covered parasympathetic and sympathetic nervous system? Working out is generally sympathetic activity. Working in refers to practices and activities you should do to balance things out on the parasympathetic side. The reason why I like this idea is that it ritualises relaxation and recovery, which many exercise enthusiasts tend to overlook.

Here's what my week might look like:

Working out:
Weightlifting 3 times a week
HIIT sprint workout once a week

Working in:
Slow mobility gym sessions 2 times a week
Daily slow breathing exercises
Long walks in nature every day
Yoga class once a week

If you map out your weekly training schedule to include both working out and working in, you're way ahead of managing your stress. And if you're feeling more stressed than usual, drop things from the Working Out side of things and stick to the Working In -activities. Movement and exercise are supposed to give you more energy throughout the day, not leave you feeling drained. Which brings us to the next topic: active recovery. I'm sure you've heard how muscles only recover at rest. But that's not entirely true. Sure, sleep is critical for muscle recovery and when you're sleeping you are definitely resting. But if you only laid in bed when you're not exercising, you wouldn't recover any better. You would recover worse. Light activity is crucial for muscle and nervous system recovery. When you're moving, you're pumping blood in and out of the muscles, shuttling in nutrients and removing waste. Active recovery falls into the working in -category. It's not a workout. Good examples include: A slow paced mobility session at the gym, yin yoga class, a long walk or even a very slow jog.

Summary:

- Stay active every day but don't just count steps, move your whole body
- Balanced muscles don't get tight or sore
- Don't engage in monotonous exercise modalities like running or biking too often
- Track your results to create intrinsic motivation
- Minimum effective dose is the right amount of exercise
- Make sure to include both working out and working in

CHAPTER 3: LOSING WEIGHT

WEIGHT LOSS

A h weight loss, an evergreen classic. Anywhere you look, the media is full of gossip on overweight celebrities, weight loss tips and success stories. It's good to keep in mind that this wasn't always the case though. Obesity was incredibly rare only a 100 years ago and the average overweight person would've qualified for a circus freak in those days. Literally. Here's what you see if you do a Google search with "circus fat man":

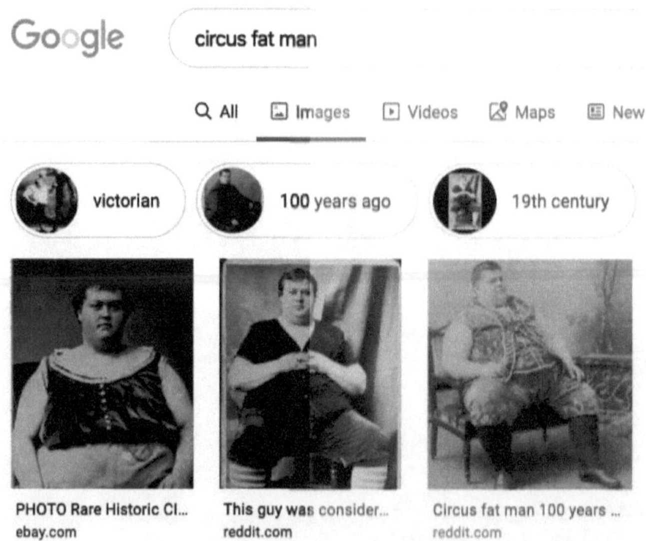

Not that bad, right? The one in the middle is Frank Williams from the 1890's and he would blend right in the modern society. Man was ahead of his time. Today we have TV shows like "My 600 lb life" because obesity is so prevalent and extreme. Now, it's important to understand that the reason I bring this up is not to mock obese people. They are victims of a sick society, and the prevalence of the obesity problem is the only proof you need. Our DNA hasn't changed in 100 years. Our environment has. When scientists want to make lab mice fat, they place them in an "obesogenic environment" where they have full access to unhealthy foods 24/7. Obesogenic environment - what a perfect term to describe our modern society. In fact, if you're not over-weight in the modern western society, you are an aberration and in the minority.

So the environment is the main problem. But we can't really change our environment, can we? Fast food is always going to be there. It will be cheap and delicious. Food marketers will find you no matter how sneaky you are. I still constantly see banner ads from a pizza chain I haven't visited in 7 years. But as with any other thing in life, we can always decide how to react to these signals. Nobody is forcing food down your throat which means you are 100% in control, always. But it sure as hell doesn't feel that way, right? We use food as a way to cheer our-selves up when we're down, as a reward when we've done some-thing good, as the centerpiece of any celebration, and so on. And then there are the cravings. Most of which are probably caused by your gut bacteria, asking you to feed them. Almost every meal becomes a struggle between giving into your temptations or staying on the right path and that can be exhausting. This is where optimizing your hormones comes in. If you create the right kind of hormonal balance in the body, you can become im-pervious to temptation. Leptin and ghrelin are in check which means you're never starving. Testosterone is high which gives you willpower and puts you back in the driver's seat. Cortisol is low which means there's no need for that piece of cake to "de-stress".

Before we jump into the "how" of losing weight, let's talk about the "why" a bit. Obviously looking subjectively better is the first thing that comes to mind. Being seriously overweight is not generally considered pretty in our current society. But beauty standards do change over time though, and most likely with the way things are going, "fat acceptance" will grow more and more popular which will surely change our perception. So maybe just focusing on social acceptance and looks isn't enough of a motivator. What about health then? Jackpot. The one thing that's common in every weight loss study ever is the fact that losing weight always improves several disease risk markers. The funny thing is that this same result tends to happen regardless of how they lost the weight. There's even a famous story of a doctor who lost weight by only eating Twinkies and some protein powder and also got healthier as a result. That for sure doesn't mean that Twinkies are healthy. It just means that being overweight is not healthy, and being of normal weight is. The Twinkie story is testament to the fact that weight loss can happen in a multitude of ways. You can lose weight by eating fast food, going vegan or paleo, by fasting (obviously) or simply increasing your exercise output. The difference is in whether it's easy and pleasurable. The Twinkie diet probably wasn't.

LOSING WEIGHT OR LOSING FAT?

Weight loss is actually a terrible term. Weight alone is really not a problem. If you're very muscular and weigh 100 kg (225 pounds), you're fine health-wise and people will compliment you on your physique. If you're not at all muscular and weigh 100 kg, you're carrying a significant amount of body fat and the situation is quite different. You will look overweight and chances are that your disease risk markers are quite high. Now the general recommendation for this person is to lose weight in any way they can: eat less and exercise more. But I would argue that the problem isn't the body weight: the problem is the ratio between muscle and fat in the body. This may sound like semantics but this is a very important distinction to make. It means that we can approach the problem from a different direction: Instead of just trying to lose weight, let's try to build more muscle. When done in a smart fashion, muscle building will also lead to a reduction in body fat. With this approach we can also forget what the scale says. Weight loss is an eventual byproduct, not the measure of immediate success. Instead we'll be tracking muscle gain and/or fat loss.

The general "calories in and calories out" model goes like this: If you eat 1500 kcal a day but burn off 2000 kcal, you will create a 500 calorie deficit and lose weight. This is sort of true and we'll get into some details later. But humans aren't physics formulas and real life tends to be messier than theory. Even if the calories in calories out -model was 100% true, you should still approach weight loss goals by looking to increase the daily burn. One pound (450g) of muscle on the body will burn approximately 50 kcal a day. Gain 10 pounds of muscle and you're burning an extra 500 kcal a day "for free". Over time this is an insane advantage. It means you can eat one additional meal every day and still end up in a calorie deficit. Or conversely, it means you don't need to run 5 miles every day, which would burn the equivalent 500 kcal.

Now regardless of whether you want to lose weight to look better or feel healthier, building more muscle will benefit you. Let's talk about looks first. A common misconception is that lifting weights will make you big and bulky. This is simply not true. Lifting weights makes you look sexy and "toned". Girls tend to get more curves, guys tend to get broader shoulders and more of a V-shape look to their body. You will only get big and bulky if you've got amazing muscle building genetics and are willing to dedicate your whole life to weight lifting. Ask any guy at the gym whether it's easy or hard to put on more muscle. Everybody who works out, knows that it's very hard to gain size. I've worked out for over 10 years and still weigh the same amount that I did when I started. I look way different, but the scale hasn't permanently moved. A muscular physique simply looks healthy and appealing and the average person who lifts weights will never look like a bodybuilder. Let's also talk about a word I've used a couple of times: toned. This is for you ladies. There is no such thing as being toned. If you got more muscle and less fat, you look toned. But there is no specific magic way of training or eating that will alone make you toned.

If your goal is health, muscles are pure magic. In fact, just very recently a group of doctors made a recommendation that muscle strength should be treated as a new vital sign. That's right, muscle strength correlates with health outcomes in the same way as your heart rate or breathing. Study after study shows that muscle strength correlates with better health outcomes, whether the researchers are measuring your ability to do push-ups, your grip strength or even just your ability to get off the floor without assistance. Losing muscle mass is also one of the main reasons why the elderly tend to get into trouble so everyone should aim to get to an old age with significant muscle mass. Even when you eventually lose some muscle, you'll still be able to get around. Muscle strength and mass are the best insurance against old age and associated health risks.

I hope I've now sold you on the idea of approaching weight loss from a different perspective. A lot of the things we'll be discussing soon will revolve around this paradigm of improving body composition, not pure weight loss.

Study link:

https://www.eurekalert.org/pub_releases/2018-10/ghn-mm-s101718.php

CALORIES IN, CALORIES OUT

As previously discussed, the general mainstream paradigm around weight loss is that you need to consume more calories than you're taking in (eating). As a scientific concept, it's relatively sound but as weight loss advice it's horrible. Some of the problems with this model include:

1. It's hard to know how many calories you're eating
2. It's hard to know how many calories you're burning
3. It's exhausting to keep track of both
4. It's so much easier to eat 300 kcal than it is to burn off 300 kcal
5. A calorie is not a calorie

1 It's hard to know how many calories you're eating

Modern technology has actually made this a bit easier than before. There are many apps that include a large variety of even packaged foods. In theory you could just look up every single thing you eat, mark it down and at the end of the day you'll know how many calories you've eaten. But even in a perfect scenario where you keep track of everything, it still gets messy. Just how much olive oil was in that restaurant salad? How many grams of meat? You get the idea. Food is not supposed to be exact science so it's hard to turn it into one.

2 It's hard to know how many calories you're burning

Again, tech helps a bit here. Most smartphones will be able to track your steps and based on your weight they can give you a rough estimate of your daily calorie burn. This is better than nothing for sure but it's still not accurate. Again, people are not physics formulas and everyone's metabolism will be different for a host of reasons. Remember that muscles burn calories even when they are not doing anything. You can take two people, same age and same weight but one has more muscle than the other. The muscular person's daily calorie burn will be higher but your smartphone doesn't know that. We'll get into the concept of slow or fast metabolism in more detail soon.

3 It's exhausting to keep track of both

Yes, calories in calories out is an insanely labor-intensive way of losing weight. You're always marking down what you're eating (or rather looking up what to eat) and comparing it to your daily burn You notice that you got 300 kcal surplus from the day and it's 9pm? Time to go on a 5 mile run. This is a very stressful way to live, and as we know, stress is going to hinder your progress.

4 It's so much easier to eat 300 kcal than it is to burn off 300 kcal

You need to run 30 minutes to burn off one Snickers bar. 300 kcal is very easy to eat. 300 kcal is a lot of work to burn off. There's just no way around this fact. If you want to live your life by the calorie counting mantra, there is nothing wrong with it. To each their own. And if you stick to it, it will work. But it won't be easy or fun. That's why I'm suggesting a different approach.

5 A calorie is not a calorie

In my mind this is the strongest argument against the calories in calories out -model. Your body doesn't treat calories equally. 100 kcal worth of Coca-Cola will elicit a completely different hormonal response than 100 kcal from broccoli. Hormones tell the body what to do at any given time and therefore it's not much of a stretch to outright say that the calories from Coca-Cola are totally different to the calories from broccoli.

DIFFERENT ENERGY SYSTEMS OF THE BODY

But Joonas, how the hell am I supposed to lose weight then if it's so hard, you say. Glad you asked. It's not hard at all. The basic problem with the premise of calories in and calories out is that it assumes that the body works in these 24 hour cycles and at the end of the day then adds or deducts weight based on the math. But that's not how the body works. Think about this concept for a second. Are you in a calorie deficit in the morning when you wake up and haven't eaten anything for 12 hours? Are you in a calorie surplus after your breakfast? Are you again in a calorie deficit after exercising? Clearly all those situations are different in terms of energy usage in the body. I will argue all day that it's possible to both build muscle and burn fat at the same time. That's what I've been doing for the past 10 years. Adding more muscle while burning fat with my weight remaining stable.

Let's look at an example day to further elaborate on the idea. Let's say you wake up in the morning after fasting for 12 hours. You have a cup of coffee and go to the gym. There you will burn maybe 200-300 kcal by lifting weights. Now at this point you've sent a signal to the body to "find" 300 kcal worth of extra energy from somewhere. As a result it's likely you've burned most of the muscle glycogen you had stored and your liver has created some extra glucose via gluconeogenesis to raise your blood sugar. You might have even used some of your own body fat for energy but since the workout was quite high tempo, most likely it was mainly driven by glycogen. When you eat 1000 kcal lunch, the body will shuttle a lot of nutrients and energy to the muscles you worked out. There is muscle damage waiting to be repaired and muscle glycogen stores waiting to be filled. Most of the carbohydrates you eat will go towards the muscles, not floating around the bloodstream. The protein and fat will be used for repair and energy. Rest of the day you'll remain active by walking around a lot and you'll have two more large meals. Walking is an ideal activity to be fueled by fat stores in the body since it's so easy and you don't need to access high demand energy systems within the muscles that would operate better with sugar. Because a lot of the energy from the food you eat will go towards muscle recovery, you'll end up burning a bit of your own body fat throughout the day for energy. You're still eating as much as you can because you want to ensure maximal muscle recovery and growth but because of such high activity you'll still probably end up in a calorie deficit. And boom, there it is: fat loss and muscle growth within the same 24 hour period.

To better understand the previous example let's take a closer look at how the body creates and uses energy. You've essentially got 3 different energy systems: the creatine-phosphocreatine system, the carbohydrate system and the fat system. The first one is the simplest, most immediate energy system. If you take a couple dozen quick running steps at full speed, you'll be using this system. But pretty quickly it runs out of energy and needs to recharge. If you wait a couple of minutes, you'll be good to go again. If instead of resting you just keep running, you'll start to use glucose for energy. It's another fast acting fuel and it will fuel your sprinting for awhile, maybe a few minutes after which your muscle glycogen stores will be depleted. At this point you'll for sure be getting tired and can't sprint as fast anymore. As you still continue jogging, your body will start shifting towards burning fat for energy. Fat stores are not as readily or easily accessible as the first two systems but they are essentially infinite. Even a very lean person will have enough body fat to keep them running for hours and hours. So sounds like fat loss is then simple, just run long enough and you'll just burn through all the fat? Well not quite. If you don't burn fat on a regular basis because you're always eating plenty of carbs, your body is not very good at burning fat. It doesn't want to do that because you've trained to avoid it. If on the other hand you don't normally eat many carbs but do engage in low level exercise often, your body will have no problems burning through its own body fat when it needs to. Your muscles can also adapt to this low glucose environment and they will start using fat more efficiently. Someone who exercises a lot but doesn't eat any carbs will be very good at fueling even those first few minutes of their sprinting with fat, either from food or from the body itself. Or to be more accurate, their body is very good at converting the fat to the form of energy they need while sprinting: glucose. Again, the body is an adaptation machine.

So it seems like a good way to burn fat is to become good at burning fat then. How do you do that? The easiest way is teaching the body to use fat for fuel. In practice this means eating less carbs but more fat. The goal initially is not to start burning through your own body fat like crazy, you just want to become good at using fat for fuel. This will ensure that when you do need to use your own body fat stores it won't become as such a shock to the body. Remember that the body wants a reason to use up those valuable stored assets. When it's good at fat burning, it will more readily release this valuable energy.

CORRECT HORMONAL ENVIRONMENT CAN MAKE ALL THE DIFFERENCE

As discussed previously, hormones signal to the body what to do at any given time. Some hormones are catabolic, meaning they encourage breaking down stuff in the body. Some are anabolic, suggesting growth. Fat burning is catabolic, muscle building is anabolic. But if you're in a catabolic state all the time you're not just burning fat, you're also breaking down muscle and other things. You also don't want to always be anabolic either as unchecked growth is not a good thing. You need a balance between the two.

Let's again look at an imaginary normal day of your average weight loss -hopeful to get an idea on how the important hormones fluctuate throughout the day:

You wake up having slept for 8 hours and fasted for 10 hours. Your cortisol will be at its natural high and growth hormone is also slightly elevated since you've been fasting for 10 hours. If you're a man, your testosterone will be high, assuming you slept well. Insulin is low. At this point you're catabolic from the cortisol but the growth hormone and testosterone will actually direct this catabolism towards the fat stores in your body, not the muscles. A good place to be if your goal is weight loss.

You eat breakfast: eggs, bacon, toast and a coffee with milk. Your cortisol will go down from the carbs in the toast and the milk but the caffeine in coffee will kick it right back up 30 minutes later once the caffeine hits you. Those same carbs will also raise your insulin and drop your growth hormone. Now you're getting anabolic: high insulin and low cortisol will direct the energy from your breakfast towards building your body. But since you haven't worked out today, there is very minimal muscle building signaling and most of the extra energy will be eventually stored as body fat. Once the caffeine hits you, you shift towards catabolism again but since your insulin is still elevated, you're not burning body fat.

You spend the morning working and drinking more coffee. The caffeine and the stressful work environment will keep your cortisol elevated for much longer than it would be naturally. You're in a catabolic state but still probably not burning fat because of the hormonal response to your breakfast.

You have lunch: tacos with beef. Similar story to what happened at breakfast but without the coffee. Carbs and the protein raise your insulin and drop your cortisol. Your growth hormone was very minimal to begin with but now you're blunting it even further again.

You have one last cup of coffee in the afternoon to get through the midday slump and work away.

After work, you go to the gym, running for 45 minutes with a steady pace on a treadmill. This actually doesn't swing your hormones too much either way. Cortisol increases a bit especially towards the end of the run as you're getting tired but it drops back down in the next couple of hours after. Human growth hormone and testosterone might go up slightly but they are just as likely to drop. Science is conflicted here which probably just means different people have different hormonal responses to steady state exercise. Exercise makes you feel good though, increasing dopamine and other feel good hormones. You're also thinking sharper after your run.

Was that good or bad? Neither. That's not the point. Food, exercise and lifestyle are not good or bad. Things just have consequences. If your goal was to burn fat or at least maintain your current weight, there are a lot of things you could have done differently to get better results. Highlights include:

- That's a lot of coffee during the day. Caffeine raises cortisol and constantly elevated cortisol will blunt the release of other useful fat burning hormones such as testosterone and growth hormone. Working is already a stressor, no need to make it more stressful with additional coffee.
- Carb timing wasn't great. You got real benefits from the carbs you had at night because they helped you to fall asleep and good sleep is always beneficial to your hormones. But during the day they also blunted the release of growth hormone pretty early in the day and created a mismatch of high insulin and high cortisol which will actually encourage fat storage, not fat burning.
- Your 45 minute run didn't really move the needle here or there in terms of fat burning. If you had done it in the morning on an empty stomach you could have capitalized on the benefits of the optimal hormonal environment and encouraged the body to burn through some of it's fat to fuel the workout.

Now let's run the same day again but just shift a few things around and cut the coffee back a bit:

- *You wake up at the same time but instead of having a full breakfast, you go for your run in the morning. Maybe a cup of coffee beforehand. You're taking advantage of the elevated corti-*

- *sol with growth hormone and testosterone and mobilizing some fat for energy.*
- *After your run, you'll head to work feeling energized and awake. Cortisol is still a bit elevated but not through the roof. Together with the endorphins and adrenaline from the work-out, it'll make you power through your morning at work.*
- *Lunch is your first meal of the day. Same lunch as previously and this time it'll work in your favor. The carbs will lower that cortisol and the insulin spike from the carbs and protein will assist in repairing some of the muscle damage from the run. Your blood sugar response to the carbs will also be lower because some of the carbs will go towards filling your muscle glycogen stores.*
- *Because you haven't taken your blood sugar on a wild ride today, you don't get that midday slump and don't feel the need to medicate with caffeine.*
- *After work you go for a nice short walk, focusing on relaxing and bringing that cortisol even further down.*
- *You finish the day in the same way as before, but for some reason you don't feel like lying down on the couch as much. Still feeling quite energetic. Maybe you go for a walk after dinner.*

Same meals, same amount of exercise but arranged a slightly different order can make a world of difference. It wasn't a dramatic lifestyle shift, you just became more aware of how you should mind your hormones, shifted a few things around and performed better as a result. That's the key to fat loss, and healthy life in general. Hormones can serve you or they can wreck you.

Now let's go one step further and look at an ideal version of the same day from a fat loss perspective. Nothing crazy, just some small additions and subtractions.

- *You wake up, have a quick cup of coffee if you feel like it and walk to work in a nice relaxed pace*
- *The walk wakes you up even if you didn't have the coffee. Since*

- *you didn't exert yourself too much, it also lowered your cortisol and made you more relaxed.*
- *You're efficiently going through your morning tasks at work and when lunch time rolls around, you head to the gym. You may or may not grab a coffee on the way to the gym, depending on how hard of a workout you're aiming for.*
- *You'll do a quick 30 minute workout with decently heavy weights. Not a brutal workout, you'll still want to feel more energized after the workout than before so you take proper rest periods but focus on moving the big muscle groups. Your growth hormone is still elevated because you haven't eaten anything and the workout will elevate it even further. Your testosterone will shoot up as a consequence of the strength training.*
- *After the workout you jump into the shower and walk back to work at a nice relaxed pace. On your way you grab lunch from the same taco place but instead of tacos you'll get a salad bowl with extra guacamole.*
- *You have your salad bowl at work and even though there's less carbs in the bowl than in the tacos, you'll still get a nice boost of insulin from the carbs and protein. This time around your body is primed to build some muscle: high insulin, high growth hormone and high testosterone all at the same time.*
- *You feel great after your lunch and keep working away. Definitely no need for that midday coffee.*
- *After work you're still feeling good so you're a bit more active than usual. You'll have more of a carb heavy or light dinner based on what you're planning to do tomorrow. If another workout is in the plans, you have a bit more carbs. If it's going to be a rest day, you take it easy on the carbs at dinner but you're not neurotic about it.*

You replaced the run with a weight lifting session and shifted the timing of some things. With these modifications you actually built some muscle and burned some fat. Your morning walk mobilized some fat stores and the midday workout and lunch pushed you straight into anabolic mode. You'll continue reaping the midday workout benefits for the next 24-48 hours depending on hard the workout was so the evening meals actually contribute either towards muscle building or fat loss depending on the amount of carbs.

Now let's dive deeper into how you should be managing your hormones for fat loss.

THE IMPACT OF DIFFERENT HORMONES

The key players when it comes to weight loss are:

- Cortisol
- Insulin
- Human growth hormone
- Testosterone
- Leptin and ghrelin
- Melatonin and vitamin D

Cortisol

As we remember from the previous chapters, cortisol is "the stress hormone". Managing cortisol is probably the most important thing when it comes to fat loss. Chronically elevated cortisol has been strongly linked to the visceral body fat, which is the worst kind. Visceral body fat means fat that's stored around important organs. Studies are pretty unanimous that visceral body fat is not good for health. It's also the least appealing looking body fat and it's got several loving nicknames: beer belly, love handles and so on.

High cortisol also blocks the secretion of several of the "good guy" hormones. For example it's borderline impossible to have high testosterone if your cortisol is always high. And cortisol can of course wreck your sleep, which will then have detrimental effects on all the other hormones.

But cortisol is not bad, per se. It's a very useful hormone. Chronically elevated cortisol is bad. The natural cycle of cortisol goes as follows: it spikes in the morning and then drops down. It'll be at its lowest at night. Cortisol will also rapidly spike when you're doing stressful activities such as working out but then it quickly drops back down. If your cortisol is flowing normally throughout the day, it's a great little ally. Only when it's being elevated too often or not allowed to drop back down is where we get into trouble.

- Only elevate cortisol when you need the energy, such as when working out and doing very intensive work
- Try to keep cortisol down as much as you can throughout the day

Cortisol elevation is essentially the same as stress. There's no need to actively bring cortisol up. It'll go up whenever you're doing anything that elevates your heart rate or engages you intensely. That's all fine and useful. Remember all the tips and tricks to managing stress from the previous chapter? Be mindful of those. Outside of your stressful activities, try to stay calm as much as possible during the day, and if something startles you, try to bring yourself back down to baseline as fast as possible after. Don't embrace stress. Try to relieve yourself from it.

Study link:

https://www.ncbi.nlm.nih.gov/pubmed/?term=visceral+fat

Insulin

Insulin is the main driver of fat storage. To over-simplify a bit: Without insulin sending the signal, your fat cells wouldn't take in fat. So it's almost impossible to gain body fat if your insulin is low. This is the key thing to understand. But insulin also drives muscle growth and other good things in the body. It's not bad, it's just very powerful.

As with cortisol, you want to elevate insulin at the right times and keep it low at other times. Fortunately this is quite easy with insulin. Carbs and protein are the only things that significantly elevate it. When do you want high insulin? When you want the body to grow. After exercising your body is primed to use insulin in muscle growth. If you haven't exercised in awhile and you spike insulin, your body will want to store the additional energy as fat.

Human Growth Hormone

Human growth hormone is quite a straightforward hormone: it says what it does and does what it says. It drives growth and cellular repair in the human body. Having higher levels of human growth hormone is basically always a good thing unless you have cancer. But it's good to understand that this doesn't mean human growth hormone causes or contributes to cancer. The very thing that makes cancer so bad is that it turns healthy processes against the body.

Human growth hormone tends to be low in overweight and obese adults. Studies have shown that treatment with human growth hormone can actually increase the effectiveness of diet in weight loss. It only makes sense that you should be trying to increase your own circulating levels of growth hormone to achieve these benefits.

Human growth hormone is obviously also a very powerful anabolic hormone and it will assist you in building muscle. Whereas insulin will promote both muscle and fat gain, human growth hormone will promote muscle gain and fat loss. It's like a miracle drug for body composition improvement. Which is why it's so common in bodybuilder and athlete circles.

So how do you go about increasing growth hormone levels naturally? Three things stand out:

1. Exercise
2. Sleep
3. Fasting

1 Exercise

But not just any exercise. Weight lifting or other high intensity forms of exercising are far superior in raising human growth hormone versus anything else. Human growth hormone signals to the body that the body needs to grow stronger to survive. Your body won't do that unless it has to. You need to send a powerful enough signal.

2 Sleep

Good quality sleep is imperative for any proper hormone function, and it's worth noting that human growth hormone gets secreted early in the night. If you go to bed late, you're missing out on this growth hormone spike.

3 Fasting

Human growth hormone continues to build as long as you don't eat. If you fast for 24 hours, studies show that your human growth hormone has gone up anywhere from hundreds to thousands of percent compared to baseline. That is truly an insane elevation and almost seems like it's too good to be true. But it makes sense: the body needs that growth hormone to build back the things it's tearing down during the fast. Once you re-feed the body uses this growth hormone rich environment to repair and rejuvenate the systems that were stressed during the fast.

Even fasting for 12 hours (for example from an 8pm dinner to 8am breakfast) is highly beneficial and fasting for 16 hours is even more powerful when it comes to burning fat.

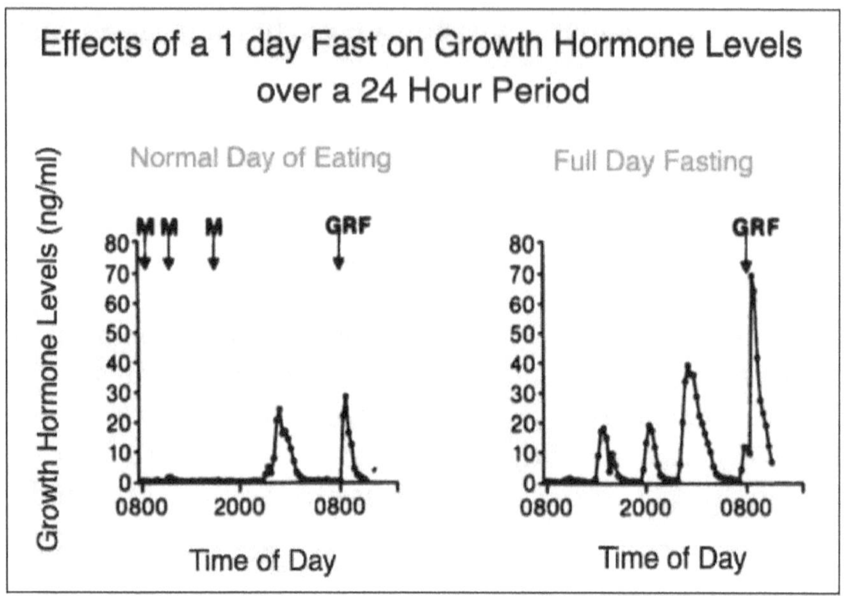

Study links:

https://www.ncbi.nlm.nih.gov/pmc/articles/PMC2435650/

https://www.ncbi.nlm.nih.gov/pmc/articles/PMC329619/

Testosterone

Testosterone builds strength, be it in the body or the mind. And remember, it doesn't matter if you're a man or a woman. You want your levels to be in the healthy range. Since testosterone strongly contributes to muscle growth, it's also very useful when it comes to weight loss. Studies show that testosterone treatment helped obese and overweight people to lose body fat, and not lean muscle, when they were calorie-deprived. That's the result you'll want as well. Remember that the goal is better body composition, not just weight loss.

Testosterone is similar to human growth hormone in the sense that high intensity exercise and sleep are the most important factors to consider. But managing your cortisol is the close third. Chronically elevated cortisol will blunt your testosterone production like nothing else. These two are strongly inversely correlated.

Study link:

https://www.ncbi.nlm.nih.gov/pmc/articles/PMC5054608/

Leptin And Ghrelin

As we remember, leptin is a satiety hormone and ghrelin is a hunger hormone.

There's really no need to get super scientific with these two. If your goal is weight loss, it's pretty clear you don't want to feel hungry all the time. The easiest way to manage hunger is to eat less carbohydrates. Carbs evoke a strong feeling of hunger (through ghrelin) whereas proteins and fats make you feel satiated (through leptin). That's not to say that carbs don't have any effect on leptin or that fats and protein wouldn't elevate ghrelin, but the effects in both cases are smaller.. Avoid carbs, embrace fats and protein.

What happens to these hormones when you combine lots of fats, protein and carbs in a single meal? Robb Wolf, the guy who wrote The Paleo Solution, tells an interesting story in his newest book Wired To Eat. There's something called The Kitchen Sink Challenge, where the contestants need to eat a literal kitchen sink full of ice cream. A guy takes on the challenge, gets about halfway through and starts struggling. A lot. He's turning green and it doesn't look like he can take another bite. His palate fatigue kicked in. Palate fatigue is a regulation mechanism (that works through leptin and ghrelin) that will essentially stop you from eating yourself to death. You just can't eat the same food until the end of time. So what does the contestant do? He orders a batch of extra salty extra crispy french fries.

He finishes the kitchen sink full of ice cream by alternating between the french fries and the ice cream. He was absolutely stuffed and he solved the problem by eating more food. But that new food was different: It had a different texture and a different flavor. With this hack he managed to override his palate fatigue. Why is this relevant to us? Think about it. What makes food so good at a great restaurant? It's the variety. Something tastes salty, something tastes sweet, some things are crunchy, others are soft. And you always have room for dessert because it's going to taste different. No wonder obesity is so prevalent. We're eating like contestants in an eating competition all the time!

It's also worth saying a couple of words about artificial sweeteners. People assume that artificial sweeteners such as those found in Diet Coke are benign for weight loss because they don't have any calories. In the strict calories in calories out -model this is true, but as we've already covered, that model does not work well in real life. Artificial sweeteners "trick" the body to think that it's eating something sweet and so the body is preparing itself for increased blood sugar. When blood sugar rises, the body releases insulin as a response. This feedback loop will ultimately make you feel full via leptin and you'll stop eating. But because artificial sweeteners don't have sugar in them, your blood sugar doesn't rise. Now you just elevated your insulin for no reason and there's no leptin secretion to make you feel full. So not only are you craving for more sweet foods because of lack of leptin, you're also unnecessarily spiking your insulin and setting the stage for fat storage. Artificial sweeteners are also linked to all kinds of unfortunate consequences such as gut bacteria dysregulation. But the bottom line is clear: you're making your fat burning lifestyle more difficult by ingesting artificial sweeteners.

Beyond diet, there is one additional thing that is very important for proper leptin and ghrelin functioning. You guessed it: It's sleep of course.

During sleep, levels of ghrelin decrease, because sleep requires far less energy than being awake does. People who don't sleep enough end up with too much ghrelin in their system, so the body thinks it's hungry and it needs more calories, and it stops burning those calories because it thinks there's a shortage.

When you don't get enough sleep, you end up with too little leptin in your body, which makes your brain think you don't have enough energy for your needs. So your brain tells you you're hungry, even though you don't actually need food at that time, and it takes steps to store the calories you eat as fat so you'll have enough energy the next time you need it. The decrease in leptin brought on by sleep deprivation can result in a constant feeling of hunger.

Melatonin And Vitamin D

No surprises here. You want to sleep when it's night time and be awake and outside when it's day time. A healthy circadian rhythm is important to all hormone functions. Look back to the chapter on sleep for tips on getting a good night's rest and make sure to get enough sun exposure during the day to raise your vitamin D levels. Or if it's the winter time, supplement with vitamin D.

LIFESTYLE PRACTICES FOR OPTIMAL HORMONAL FUNCTION

Based on the previous examples, we can now recognize some general recommendations on how you should live your life if your goal is to burn fat.

Overall Health

First and foremost: follow the recommendations laid out on chapter 1 on overall health. Maintain a good sleep schedule, fast regularly for 12 to 16 hours every day (night), eat natural whole foods, manage your stress, stay active and exercise. You'll be setting the stage for optimal hormonal function.

Diet

Keep your ghrelin and leptin in check by eating a generally low carb diet. Low carb can mean anything from 0 to 150 grams of carbs every day depending on your activity levels, your insulin sensitivity, your age and your ancestry. Try different approaches and see what makes you feel the best. If you have a lot of weight to lose or don't do well on carbs, consider trying out a ketogenic approach where you eat almost no carbs. You can find tons and tons of info on low carb and ketogenic diets online.

If and when you do eat carbs, eat them around your workouts. Either a bit before or a bit after. That way you're setting the stage for muscle growth, not fat storage. Remember everything we've talked about insulin? Play around with both of these approaches and see which one feels better. Personally I prefer working out on an empty stomach and having my carbs after. But you might feel different. The amount of carbs is again something that you need to figure out for yourself. If you're making progress, losing fat and/or getting stronger, you're in a good place. If you're not getting stronger, you might want to increase the carbs around the workouts a bit. If you're not burning fat, you might want to try reducing the carbs. Play around with them and have fun.

Don't worry about counting calories but in the beginning it might be helpful to pay some attention to them. For example try to calculate how many calories you normally eat right now without changing anything and then compare what a day of low carb eating looks like. You'll get some idea on how much you're consuming. The key thing is to avoid going massively over or under. If previously you were eating 3000 kcal a day and now you're only eating 1500 kcal, that's a huge difference and over time it will cause you problems. Low carbs foods are very satieting and it's easy to undereat. But once you understand how many calories you're approximately getting, don't sweat it. You'll quickly build up an understanding that you need to eat maybe 3 meals a day to hit a decent caloric level. Just keep eating 3 meals per day and forget about the calorie counting.

The problem with a severe calorie deficit is that over time it will start working against your goals. Your metabolism will slow down and the 1500 kcal a day -pace will become your new normal. Your body will adapt to it. You'll still want to be able to enjoy life and go wild with food every now and then, so you'll want to maintain a good active metabolism. Train the body to use the energy it's getting. You can't build muscle if you're not eating enough. And our strategy is to increase muscle and burn fat.

Exercise

Regularly engage in high intensity exercise. If you're starting from 0, go easy in the beginning. For someone who has very little workout experience, 2 days a week is a good place to start. Slowly build up to 3 or 4 but that's enough. Working out will boost your testosterone and growth hormone but keep in mind that rest and recovery is even more important to keep these strength builders working full time.

Choose an exercise modality you like. If you find group classes motivating, consider crossfit or something similar. If you prefer working out alone, get a gym membership. If you have money to spend, a personal trainer can be a very good investment. You'll want to learn how to train the right way. But a personal trainer is by no means a necessity. There are great workout formulas for beginners but in my mind one stands heads and shoulders above the rest: 5x5 Stronglifts. It's a super simple gym program where you do two different workouts: workout A and workout B. You'll alternate between these two until the end of time. You'll only be doing the big main lifts: squats, deadlifts, overhead presses, bench presses and barbell rows. It will build strength and muscle very fast. There is even a great app you can use which will automatically track your workouts and teach you the movements. I can't recommend it enough. If you're a more advanced lifter or just want to learn more, read the following chapter regarding muscle gains and consider switching to a more advanced lifting program at some point. But seriously, 5x5 Stronglifts is a great place to start for anyone. Google it.

If you only absolutely love running and nothing else, and I haven't been able to talk you out of it yet, consider at least alternating your running modalities. Consistent long distance running will only make you more efficient at running. You'll start to burn less and less calories when running, your body will sacrifice unnecessary muscle mass and your metabolism will slow down. One or two days a week do sprints, full speed for 30 seconds followed by a 3-5 minute rest. After 5 sprints you're done. And maybe next time sprint shorter distances. Or up a hill. Maybe even a bit longer ones on occasion. Sometimes head out for a light jog. Some days go for a bit longer, faster run. Keep it interesting.

WHAT ABOUT SUPPLEMENTS?

The market is full of all kinds of weight loss supplements. As a general rule of thumb: they are all bullcrap. That's not to say they don't work. Some of them might. But the effects are minimal compared to all the important things we've been talking about: diet, sleep, exercise. Don't waste your money.

Now, if you're deficient in crucial vitamins and minerals, supplementing can be a good idea. If you're eating a good variety of natural foods, chances are your bases are covered. But consider testing your vitamin & mineral levels at some point in your life. It's going to cost a bit but think about it in the same way as your car maintenance. You have no problem spending a few hundred dollars or euros a year to keep your car running fine. Why wouldn't you perform a similar check under the hood with your meat machine? You can always buy a new car. You can't buy a new body.

And if you're vegan, then definitely supplement with vitamin B12 and DHA (An omega 3 fatty acid found in marine organisms).

HACKS AND TWEAKS

Actually there aren't any hacks to be found here. I hate health hacks. You can't hack your way to better health. You for sure can hack your way to losing weight quickly but not in a sustainable healthy fashion. So let's call these following tips tweaks. They are relatively minor lifestyle habits that will further help you get towards your goals, but they aren't necessary by any means.

Longer Fasts (24 Hours And Up)

Especially if you still have gut issues after eating whole real foods and following all the lifestyle advice we've covered, longer fasts might be a magic cure for you. Personally I've experimented with longer fasts for a few years now. I've done a 5 day water fast three times, 5 day fasting mimicking diet twice, dozens of 24 hour fasts and I've now landed on my sweet spot: I water fast for 3 days once per quarter, 4 times a year. And for me it works like magic. My gut always feels fantastic after every fast and the effects last for a long time. The reasons behind the healing effects of fasting are still being studied but a couple of things are clear: Fasting increases autophagy and releases stem cells. Autophagy literally translates to self-eating and that makes sense. When you're not eating food, you're eating yourself. Why is this a good thing? Because the body is smart. It will eat poorly functioning cells first. Autophagy that happens during fasting is like spring cleaning. The body gets rid of unnecessary gunk and rebuilds brand new cells once you stop the fast and start eating. This rebuilding happens through the aforementioned increased stem cells and the hugely elevated human growth hormone. Stem cells are sort of the building blocks of life: They can become any cell in your body. They are the raw material that builds your organs, your immune system, even your brain. Stem cell transplants can cost tens of thousands of dollars. Fasting is literally free.

Water fasting is just that: You're only consuming water and maybe some other non-caloric substances like coffee or tea. It's good to supplement with mineral or sea salt during fasting to avoid getting dehydrated. I've personally used between 5-10 grams of Himalayan salt every day. I mix into the water I drink throughout the day. Another good option is to opt for good quality sparkling water that has calcium, magnesium, potassium and sodium in it. Don't push yourself during fasts but stay active. Go for walks, do some dynamic stretching or yoga. Work on projects. You've got an amazing amount of extra free time when you're not planning meals, buying food, cooking, eating and washing dishes. Fasting will also teach you a lot about your relationship with food. Does watching Netflix without a plate in front of you feel boring? Good, you identified a blindspot in your life. It's not a good idea to just mindlessly consume food when focusing on what's happening on TV. When you start eating again stay mindful of the things you noticed during the fast. Having regular access to delicious food is an amazing thing and meals are meant to be enjoyed.

Now, here's the most important thing: Even though longer fasts will burn plenty of fat, that's not the reason to fast. Fasting is a health-promoting tool first and foremost. Fasts will promote good hormone balance but if you're heavily hormonally compromised going into a fast, you might create more problems. And don't start with a 3 or a 5 day fast. Try a 24 hour fast. If that feels easy, push for 36 or 40 hours. Slowly build up to 3 days. And don't fast too often, the magic happens after the fact when your body starts re-building. In a very real sense, you also need to recover from fasting.

Omega 3 / Omega 6 Fatty Acid Balance

There's a lot of stuff we don't know about the ancient human diet but few things are undebatable. One thing that's especially interesting is the ratio between Omega3 and Omega3 fatty acids. In a modern western diet, we get way more Omega6 than Omega3. The ratio can be something along the lines of 20:1. Ancient humans were closer to 2:1 or even 1:1. Omega3 fatty acids are generally anti-inflammatory whereas Omega6's are inflammatory. This is an oversimplification, because Omega6's are also necessary. But the ratio between the fatty acids is important for keeping the body in balance. Too much inflammation will hamper your ability to recover, burn fat and build muscle. Omega3 supplementation has been shown to lower cortisol and contribute to lean muscle gains and improved body composition.

Omega3's are mainly found in fish whereas Omega6's are everywhere. But even large land mammals like cows, when pasture raised, will have way more Omega3's than industrially raised grain-fed animals. To fix your Omega3/Omega6 -balance your should therefore focus on two things:

- Avoid industrially raised meat when you can. Choose mainly organic and pasture-raised meat, or even wild game if you can
- Eat fatty fish like salmon, but the same rules apply here. Wild caught fish will have more Omega3's than industrially grown fish.

Sauna Use

Saunas are great for several reasons. You sweat out toxins, work out your cardiovascular system and let off some steam both figuratively and literally. Elevated body heat and the cooldown that happens after will make you more relaxed and can make you sleep better. In Finland, where I'm from, saunas are very common. In fact there are more saunas than people in Finland, and almost every apartment will have their own sauna. This makes studying the benefits of regular sauna use quite easy and most sauna studies therefore originate from Finland. Regular sauna use has been shown to reduce all-cause mortality by a staggering 40% in men who used the sauna 5-7 times a week.

There is one major hormonal impact which especially makes sauna use something to consider, and what probably contributes to the aforementioned mortality reduction: They can raise human growth hormone significantly. Two 20-minute sessions a day at 80 celsius can result in a 2-fold increase of HGH over baseline. And the benefits stack up even further if you increase exposure. Hit the sauna after your workouts, if your gym has one.

Study link:

https://bmcmedicine.biomedcentral.com/articles/10.1186/s12916-018-1198-0

Cold Exposure

Like heat, cold exposure can also have a powerful impact on the body. Cold exposure refers to things like cold showers, cryotherapy and cold water immersion. The studies on testosterone and growth hormone aren't clear on the results but a couple of things that do seem pretty bulletproof: Cold exposure improves your immune function and lowers stress. As we know, stress will kill your gains and in many ways and anything that will improve stress tolerance is worth considering. Improved immune function is of course very beneficial as well. When you get sick less often, you'll stay on track easier.

One additional benefit of cold exposure seems to be improved sleep. Anecdotally, taking cold showers late in the evening has had a tremendously positive effect on my sleep quality. I know cold showers can sound a bit scary but remember that your body is an adaptation machine. You'll very quickly build tolerance to the cold, and what made you shiver a few days ago is a breeze today.

One thing to note: Don't buy into the hype of expensive cryotherapy centers. You can get the same benefits (or very close at least) very easily with cold showers and cold water immersion.

CLOSING WORDS

You might have heard about The Conscious Competence Ladder. This is what it looks like:

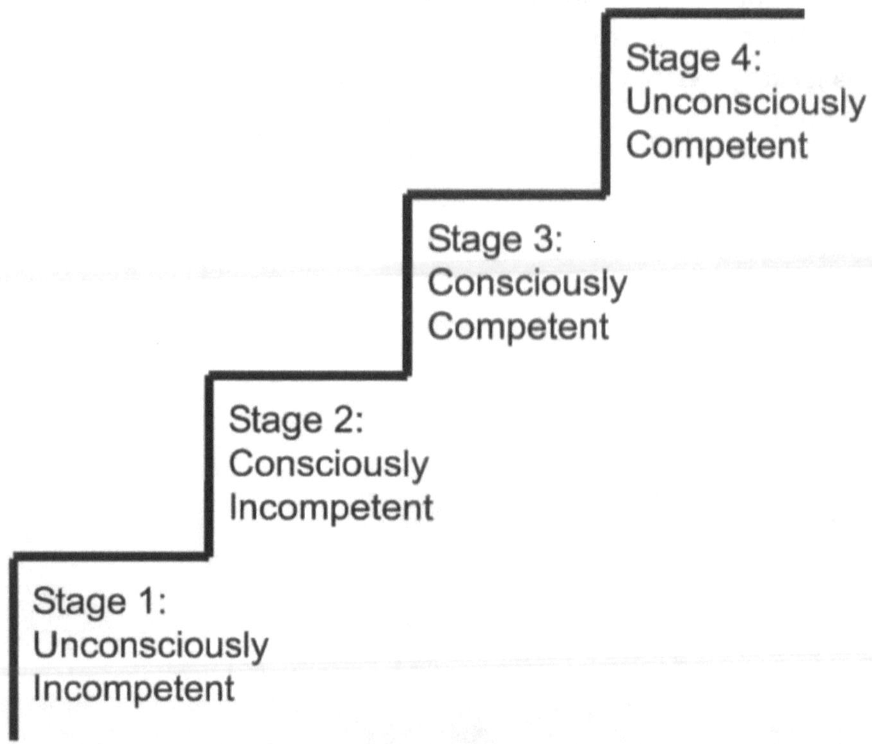

Any time you're doing something totally new, you start at level 1. You are unconsciously incompetent. You don't yet know that you don't know anything. Maybe this is you when it comes to hormones. Maybe previously you had no idea what they were or what they did. After reading this book you'll probably feel like level 2. You now know that you don't know much. But once you start applying the advice to your life you'll quickly graduate to level 3. It takes work to manage your hormones but you're well aware of how your lifestyle impacts them. Before you know it, this new lifestyle becomes second nature to you and graduate to level 4. You just intuitively do the right thing and suddenly everything is easy.

Remember that even though fat loss can happen quite fast in the beginning, you're not in it for the short term results. You want to transform your body and stay that way. You want to get to level 4. The reward from changing your lifestyle isn't ultimately going back to your old lifestyle with a new body. The reward is the new body and the maintenance fee for that meat machine is your new lifestyle. Take care of your body because you love it and enjoy the ride.

CHAPTER 4: GAINING STRENGTH AND MUSCLE

BODYBUILDING?

Let's make one thing clear at the start. This is not a bodybuilding guide. Bodybuilding is at the ultimate end of the spectrum of gaining muscle, and therefore not a healthy pursuit. Nothing is healthy when taken to an extreme. I'm not a massive guy myself, and most people aren't willing to do what it takes to get truly huge. I'm personally mainly interested in strength and performance. And looking better is just a nice side effect. If you're already an experienced lifter and your goal is to get absolutely massive, you're in a very small minority. This book is meant for the masses and the everyday person. It's a summary of what I wished I knew 10 years ago. But even if you are an experienced lifter, unless you're already very well versed in the role of hormones when it comes to muscle gains, and more importantly how to manage those hormones, stick around because you might just learn something new.

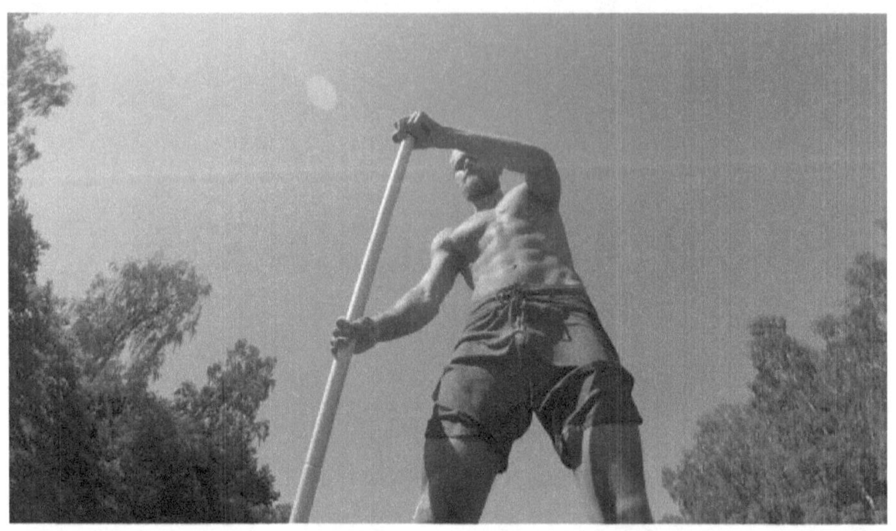

Obligatory topless picture of the author to convince the reader that they know something about the subject matter

MUSCLE AND STRENGTH 101

In theory I suppose almost everyone knows the basic mainstream principles of muscle growth: damage the muscles by exercising hard and they respond by getting bigger and stronger if you eat enough food. There is truth in this but like the "calories in calories out" model we've previously discussed, it's a gross oversimplification of the process. Remember the study about the people who built more muscle by taking anabolic steroids and not exercising, than the people who exercised? Clearly hormones are the key when it comes to muscle gains. You should therefore build your strength training program with hormones in mind. Using big muscle groups will raise your testosterone and growth hormone the most, and that means that big lifts such as squats and deadlifts are more useful in elevating these hormones than bicep curls.

Muscles themselves are dumb machines. They don't know anything. They just do what the central nervous system (CNS) tells them to do. CNS tells them to contract and they contract. CNS tells them to release and they release. A great analogy I learned from the MindPump podcast: Think of your muscles as the speakers and the central nervous system as the amplifier. Speakers don't play any tunes without the amplifier and even the most powerful speakers become puny if the amp is weak. And vice versa. Strength is a mixture of having a powerful amplifier, your CNS, and powerful speakers, your muscles.

Muscle size is part of getting stronger but not the whole picture. If you have very dense smaller muscles, you might still be stronger than a guy with bigger bubbly muscles. Most people will still want to gain size because let's face it, big muscles tend to look good. But it's important to understand that you can tailor your regiment to either get you bigger, or shredded. And the best thing for most people is to alternate between these two.

Muscles can get bigger through a couple of modalities: sarcoplasmic hypertrophy and myofibrillar hypertrophy. Let's break these word monsters down a bit.

Sarcoplasmic hypertrophy refers to muscle glycogen storage growth. Simply put it means your muscles will adapt to store more energy in the form of carbohydrates inside them.

Myofibrillar hypertrophy refers to actual muscle cell components increasing in number. The size gains aren't as big as with sarcoplasmic hypertrophy but whereas sarcoplasmic hypertrophy mainly contributes to muscle size, myofibrillar hypertrophy actually makes the muscles stronger.

To avoid using big words all the time, let's use another analogy. If your muscle is a car, sarcoplasmic hypertrophy refers to building a bigger gas tank within the muscles and myofibrillar hypertrophy means building a bigger engine. Both will make the car look bigger but the potential for the gas tank to grow in size is bigger than the engine. Makes sense?

You can be very strong and still have small gas tanks in the muscles because (in the car analogy) you don't need a lot of gas to go very fast for a short distance. That's why olympic power-lifters will focus more on the myofibrillar side of things and as a result aren't as big as bodybuilders who mainly focus on building a bigger gas tank. But the engines in bodybuilders muscles usually aren't as big and powerful as with olympic powerlifters.

Now the average person should include both these modalities

in their training and the reason is simple: newbie gains.

Study link:

https://www.ncbi.nlm.nih.gov/pubmed/8637535

WAIT, DID YOU JUST CALL ME A NEWBIE?

Ah, newbie gains, one of my favorite concepts in life. As we've established, the body is an adaptation machine. Whenever you do anything, your body will try to quickly adapt to get better at it. Those adaptations are quick and powerful. This means that the best way to shape and mold the body to a favorable direction is to switch between different adaptations often enough to constantly enjoy the benefits of newbie gains.

The name newbie gains comes from the quick muscle gains "newbies" (people who have never worked out) tend to make in the gym. But that quick progress will inevitably slow down. It's easy and quick to get decently strong. It's very hard and time consuming to get really strong. It's easy and quick to build some size in your muscles. It's very hard and time consuming to build really big muscles.

The concept of newbie gains will be at the center of my training recommendations. You should focus on a specific adaptation for some time and then switch to a different one. Focus on the new one for some time and then switch back or towards something new. In this way you're always sending a powerful signal to your body, asking it to change and become better.

There are three things you can focus on with your strength training:

1. Central nervous system strength
2. Bigger gas tanks within the muscles

3. Bigger engines within the muscles

Before we jump into more detail on each modality, let's cover some basic terms. A set refers to a single set of an exercise. A set might consist anywhere between 1 to 30 repetitions of that exercise. Rest period means the amount of time you'll be resting between the sets.

TRAINING THE CENTRAL NERVOUS SYSTEM STRENGTH

Everyone should aim to have a strong central nervous system. In the context of muscle and strength CNS strength refers to your ability to recruit the maximum amount of muscle fibers to accomplish a specific task. CNS doesn't directly have anything to do with the muscles themselves. It's a neurological system that connects to the muscles via nerves. Therefore having a strong central nervous system is almost the same thing as having a strong brain. Biologically CNS refers to a larger whole than the brain, but the brain drives the processes.

CNS is the most important component of strength. If your CNS is not working properly, you can't use your muscles properly. Therefore taking care of your CNS should be your number one priority when it comes to strength training but also a healthy lifestyle in general. Remember that muscle strength is nowadays being viewed as a vital sign that can actually diagnose your disease risk.

On a conceptual level, training the CNS is quite simple: Ask the body to recruit the muscle fibers often enough and it will obey and become better at this task. Heavy strength training is superior to lighter lifting when it comes to CNS activation. But here's where it gets complicated: Chances are you're not very good at activating all your muscles. If you have any aches, pains or tightness, it's because your CNS connection to your muscles isn't working optimally. If you just ask the CNS to work hard but the connection to the muscles isn't good, you'll end up recruiting the load unevenly. This will raise your risk of injury and over time will create an unbalanced physique.

The reason why I'm quite sure that you don't have a very good muscle connection at the moment is simple: Almost everyone in the modern society has tightness and pain somewhere sometimes. It's because our bodies have adapted to a lifestyle where you don't move often enough and with enough variety. When I'm writing this book right now my left rhomboid (a muscle in the upper back) is getting tighter and tighter. Nobody's perfect.

Fortunately training this mind muscle connection is quite simple: Let's say I'm going to the gym after I'm done writing and I'm aware that my left rhomboid is tight. Before I lift heavy, I'll make sure to go through my main muscle groups to activate them, especially the rhomboids. Activating the muscles simply means practicing the movements with minimal load beforehand. For the rhomboids, I'll grab a rubber band, hook it onto something and will do a couple of sets of light rows where I'm really focusing on squeezing the rhomboids and working the muscles through their full range of motion. But the rhomboid tightness is definitely linked to overactive or tight muscles somewhere else in the body so I won't stop there. I'll also work my chest, my shoulders, my hips and my knees and ankles. When I'm feeling nice and loose, I'll start to load the muscles with weight. Because I did all this prepwork, which really only took me 10 minutes, I'm now recruiting the muscles fully when I work out. Less aches and pains in the future and more balanced muscle development.

After my prepwork when I now lift heavy, I'm engaging the entire central nervous system. The lifts that target the central nervous system the most are the big powerful multi joint movements such as deadlifts and squats. In fact, the first heavy deadlift is usually a memorable experience to anyone. For most people it's the first time in their lives they have ever worked as hard. The feeling is an interesting combination of panic and full unwavering focus. "Can I really lift this? Yes I can!" That's the stuff that'll make you stronger. Getting out of your comfort zone and asking the body to work harder than it's ever worked before. It's also very taxing for the central nervous system and shouldn't be done too often. But more on that later.

TRAINING FOR BIGGER GAS TANKS WITHIN THE MUSCLES

This area is where bodybuilders tend to spend most of their training time as bigger gas tanks equal bigger muscles. If you've ever seen a pro bodybuilder working out, you'll know they often do it with smaller weights than you might expect someone of that size to do. But the sets are long: 8 to 15 repetitions or even longer. At the end of their workout they might do very long sets with very little rest, aiming to get a massive pump. The pump refers to pumping the muscles full of blood. As you can imagine, big muscles all pumped up will look very impressive. The pump is however fleeting and after a few hours their muscles will get back to their normal size.

Studies show that working in the 8 - 12 repetition range will cause the most sarcoplasmic hypertrophy, meaning it will create a bigger gas tank. Rest periods between sets are usually between 45-90 seconds. Essentially you'll be depleting the muscles of gas, carbohydrates, with every set, giving the body some time to replenish the tank and then doing it again. Because you're not allowing the body to fully replenish the tank, your body will want to build a bigger tank for next time. It doesn't like running dry.

Higher rep ranges, 12-30 will create a bigger pump. When working on a pump, you only give the muscles minimal rest between sets. 15-45 seconds. This is not enough time for the body to fill the tank or even expel the waste products from the muscles, you're just pumping more and more blood into them. It sounds bad but there are always some benefits to forcing the body to work hard. And here it's pulling out all the stops to keep those muscles moving, desperately pumping more blood and nutrients into the muscles. The research actually isn't all that clear on how the pump assists in muscle growth but studies do show that it does. So there's benefit in aiming to get a pump even if you're not going to the beach right after.

Rep ranges that are too high, usually anything over 30 will not really contribute to muscle growth anymore. They turn into conditioning workouts. As a rule of thumb: if you can do over 30 reps, you're using weights that are too light. Go heavier.

Study links:

https://www.ncbi.nlm.nih.gov/pubmed/31166954

https://www.researchgate.net/publication/285754036_The_Muscle_Pump_Potential_Mechanisms_and_Applications_for_Enhancing_Hypertrophic_Adaptations

TRAINING FOR BIGGER ENGINES WITHIN THE MUSCLES

Olympic powerlifters tend to focus on building strong engines rather than huge gas tanks. They'll mainly work with very short sets, anywhere between 1 to 5 repetitions, and have long rest periods in between the sets. Minimum 3 minutes, usually even longer. The goal here is to exert maximum amount of force for a very short time, and then rest long enough for the energy systems within the body to rebound back to baseline. Whereas sarcoplasmic hypertrophy, gas tank training, uses mainly the carbohydrate stores within the muscles, myofibrillar hypertrophy, engine training, uses the creatine-phosphocreatine system. As you remember, different energy systems were covered in the weight loss chapter. Creatine-phosphocreatine system is very powerful but runs out of gas quickly. When training that system, the sets can't last very long. After a short while, anywhere between 15-30 seconds, you run out of energy and the body will switch to burning carbohydrates. Keep it short.

Your muscles will replenish the creatine-phosphocreatine stores fairly quickly, usually between 3 to 5 minutes, depending on how hard you worked them. To train the muscle engines therefore you should be working in the 1-5 rep range and resting at least 3 minutes between every set.

As with gas tank training, there are a couple of different modalities when it comes to training the muscle engines: strength and power. Strength refers to your raw ability to move heavy weight. When you're really grinding it out. Power refers to the ability to exert force rapidly and explosively. A good example of strength is a slow heavy deadlift. A good example of power training is a jumping squat where you squat all the way down and explosively jump up.

Regardless of whether you're training for strength or power, the same basic principles still apply: Short bursts of all out effort followed by a long rest period. The long rest period is key: If you aren't fully recovered from your last set, you'll be training the gas tank, not the engine.

This type of training is especially good at building new mitochondria within the muscles and to some extent the effect is systematic, meaning that the rest of the body benefits as well. Mitochondria are the power plants of cells. They create adenosine triphosphate, ATP, which is the energy currency of all life. Within muscles more mitochondria equals more power. Mitochondrial dysfunction is linked to many disease states so taking care of your mitochondria is smart for overall health. Lots of well functioning mitochondria equals better overall health.

The important anabolic hormones testosterone and human growth hormone tend to respond the best to this type of strength & power -focused training. All kinds of resistance training will elevate them but the exercises that elevate especially testosterone the most tend to be big explosive movements. It makes sense especially if you think about it from an evolutionary perspective: the only time an animal needs to engage in explosive powerful movements is when it's a matter of life and death. The body will call upon every possible reserve to ensure survival.

High intensity interval training, or HIIT for short, should also fall in this category, but HIIT is often misunderstood and abused. People will usually engage in HIIT training with rep ranges and rest periods that look like gas tank training when really they should be focusing on the engine. A good example, box jumps: You often see people doing tons and tons of box jumps in the gym until they are exhausted. This is just plain dumb. The benefit of a box jump is in training the body to explode off the ground rapidly. You do that a few times and then you rest long enough to do it again with maximum force. You do it 20 times and now you're just beating yourself up for no reason. Same thing with running sprints. If you can sprint for longer than 30 seconds, you're doing it wrong. When you sprint at full speed, 30 seconds is an eternity. You should sprint with maximum speed until your speed starts to drop and stop there. For most people this happens in less than 30 seconds. And if you're not resting for 3 minutes or more between sprints, you're doing it wrong and just beating yourself up again. Stuff like that should only be reserved for a competition situation. It shouldn't really be a part of training.

FUELING YOUR TRAINING

The fitness industry and food marketers probably have you convinced of two things: that you need to eat tons of protein and that you should do it in the form of protein bars and shakes. Protein has long been marketed as a magical macronutrient that you just can't get enough of and it's added to everything to make things appear more healthy. Protein yoghurt! Protein milk! Protein pancakes! As with most of these mainstream health "truths", this one is also bullcrap. First of all, the word 'protein' means a lot of things. Snake venom is a protein. You probably don't want that added to your pancakes. Some forms of protein are more anabolic than others, it all depends on their amino acid profile. Animal-based proteins are the clear winners here but there are some pretty good plant-based protein sources as well. If you're vegan, you might want to consider using hemp protein or a protein mix that has a lot of different plant proteins in it.

Studies show that a sufficient level of protein intake for muscle growth is actually quite low, in between 50-100g per day depending on your weight and muscle mass. If you eat meat or eggs daily, you're most likely getting enough protein. If you eat meat with every meal, you're definitely getting enough unless you're a high level strength or bodybuilding athlete. The potential extra protein from protein bars and shakes is not necessarily bad for you, but it's not important either. What is bad for you however is the other crap in those bars and shakes: artificial sweeteners, emulsifiers and other low quality processed garbage. Skip the bars and shakes, stick to whole natural foods.

There's also the myth of the post-workout shake. The theory goes as follows: If you consume protein immediately after the workout, it will go straight to the muscles and assist their recovery and boost their growth. There might be some theoretical truth there but even if there is, the difference between having a shake immediately after a workout vs having a meal one hour after a workout will be minimal. And actually, hormonally there's a really good reason to wait a bit after a workout before you eat. As we've learned so far, human growth hormone gets elevated both from working out and fasting. When you eat, it drops. If you wait a bit before you eat, your growth hormone will keep building up and when you do eat, you'll be in more of an anabolic state.

So a sufficient amount of protein is necessary but that amount is fairly easy to acquire from normal whole foods. What about carbs and fats then? Here's where it gets a bit more complicated. As you might remember from the gut health chapter, different people should have different carb and fat intake. Some people are really good at using carbs and they can get away with way more. Some people don't do well with a high carb intake and they shouldn't eat high-carb even if they are exercising a lot. As a general rule training the central nervous system and the muscle engines are well suited for a low carb intake. Training the muscle gas tanks might be harder if you aren't eating a lot of carbs. But that doesn't mean that you can't do it. You should just back down on the weights a bit and not push yourself super hard. Someone who can eat tons of carbs can push their gas tank training a bit harder. In this way your ability to handle carbohydrates is actually probably the single biggest factor in your ability to get bigger.

Personally I'm a bit screwed here. My stomach gets messed up when I eat a lot of carbs so I don't feel it's worth it to try to push the carb intake higher just to get bigger. But then again my little brother, who has almost the same genes as me, eats lots of carbs, works out the same way and is pretty much the same size as me. Carbs aren't magic either. Speaking of brothers, the youngest one is also an interesting case to bring up. Every male in my family was naturally skinny as a kid, including the youngest. But he started lifting weights at 17. And because the internet was around and information was easy to find, he actually followed some pretty good diet and exercise advice from the start, unlike my generation who just relied on random advice from the meatheads at the gym. And he blew up, weighing almost 100 kg at 20 where as me and my other brother really struggle to get past 75 kg. You know what's the difference? Hormones. The insulin sensitivity, growth hormone and testosterone potential of a 17 year old is insane compared to someone in their 20s, 30s or older. The younger you start, the easier all this stuff is. If you're not working out, start today, not tomorrow.

Back to carbs and fats. You might remember from the gut health chapter that people who eat low carb will actually get better at using fat to fuel their muscles directly. If you eat low carb and exercise regularly, your muscles will get better at using fat for fuel and won't need as much glycogen. The mitochondria within the cells will adapt to this new energy environment and over time you'll start to foster a community of new fat-eating mitochondria instead of carb consuming mitochondria you had previously. A low carber's performance might therefore be similar or better to a high carber, but the high carber will always have an edge when it comes to muscle size.

Another reason why a higher carb diet is beneficial in putting on size is of course the hormone insulin. As we remember, insulin makes things grow and that is true for both muscle and fat. A high carber will be spiking their insulin regularly, setting the stage for growth. If you don't eat a lot of carbs, this is where strategic spiking of insulin comes in though. As a low carber, aim to eat the little carbs you do eat mainly around your workouts to spike the insulin when it serves you the most. Note that if you don't feel good consuming lots of carbs, don't. You won't build more muscle if you're getting unhealthy in the process. Know your body and work with it, not around it.

Then there's the question on when you should eat in terms of your workout. There are some theoretical differences when it comes to hormone balance with different scenarios. But in all honesty you should probably do what you like the most and what is realistic to your schedules. I personally prefer working out on an empty stomach. Growth hormone is already high from the night before and I just feel at my sharpest then. Most people will probably prefer to eat something before or even during their workouts. Play around with different timings and see what serves you the best. As long as you're doing everything else right, meal or workout timing won't make a huge difference either way.

Somewhat unintuitively, intermittent fasting is an awesome tool for muscle building. Intermittent fasting refers to relatively short fasts every day. Anywhere from 12 to 18 hours. As you remember, human growth hormone goes up when you're fasting. HGH is your best friend when it comes to muscle gains and therefore keeping it up should be one of your biggest priorities. Now obviously when you fast for let's say 16 hours every day, you'll only be eating in a window of 8 hours. You need to eat a lot during these 8 hours to get enough energy to grow. But all that feeding then happens in a tremendously anabolic environment where HGH is high. Intermittent fasting is the easiest and most powerful natural way to bump up your HGH. Trust me, higher levels of human growth hormone are worth skipping breakfast over. And remember, any calories will break a fast. Even a bit of milk in your morning coffee. To get the full hormonal benefits of intermittent fasting, only consume calories within your feeding window.

Study link:

https://www.ncbi.nlm.nih.gov/pmc/articles/PMC6566799/

TRAINING REGIMEN FOR OPTIMAL HORMONE BALANCE

So with all that said, how and how often should you then train for muscle size and strength? You should alternate between different target adaptations but practice each of them long enough to see results. Let's keep it simple: one adaptation per month. This month you'll focus on strength, next month a bigger gas tank, then getting a pump, then power, then rotating back to strength and so on. Some of these phases will have a bigger impact on hormones than others. Strength and power training will elevate testosterone and growth hormone more than gas tank or pump training. But since you'll be alternating between these modalities, you'll be going into your gas tank and pump sessions with high baseline levels from the previous month and thus reaping their benefits.

You should train the whole body every time you work out. The reason for that is that you'll want to hit each muscle group several times a week. When you work out your chest for example, you send a signal to the body that it needs to adapt and build muscle. Local muscle protein synthesis in the chest muscles will be elevated for the next 24-48 hours and but then it will drop down to almost baseline. In practice after two days your body is no longer building muscle in your chest. So now you're ready to work out again and spike the signal for another 24-48 hours. Most gym programs you find online or hear about from bros at the gym are so called body part splits. In a body part split you'll for example hit chest on monday, back on wednesday, legs on friday and arms on saturday. In the context of the muscle building signal only lasting for a couple of days, a body part split is then pretty inefficient. Most of the week you're not building any muscle in any given body part. But with a full body program done 3 times a week, the signal is always on so to speak.

A full body program is also superior in terms of hormone impact. Studies are quite clear on the fact that mobilizing the large muscle groups will spike testosterone and human growth hormone more than working on small muscles. Since you'll be hitting those large muscle groups with every workout, you'll have higher hormone levels and build more muscle as a result. Each full body workout should include some sort of leg exercise such as squatting or deadlifting, a pushing exercise such as bench press or overhead press, a pulling exercise such as pull-ups or rows and a core exercise like a side chop or hanging knee raises. That's it, no need to get fancy unless you've been doing this for awhile and have specific muscles you especially want to target.

When you are working the whole body every time, you need to be mindful not to beat yourself up. Your weekly exercise volume will be high even if you're only doing one movement per body part every time you work out. Try to avoid lifting to failure. Lifting to failure means that you simply can't get the weight up anymore. When you lift to failure, you're creating a lot of stress for the muscle and the central nervous system. You'll need a long time to recover from extreme exertions like this and you won't be good to go again in a couple of days. Leave some gas in the tank and stop a couple of reps before failure. In practice this means that if you can do 7 reps with a given weight, don't do more than 5. Manage your weights accordingly, don't just push the weights higher all the time. Minimum effective dose.

Range of motion is also an important concept to cover. Often in the gym you see people doing so called partial exercises: They squat a bit down but not all the way. Or they drop the dumbbells a shoulder level but not all the way to chest level when doing overhead presses. Yeah you can move more weight around when you're cheating like this but you're not doing yourself any favors. Full range of motion exercises will build more muscle than partials. You might need to lower the weights a bit but it's worth the ego hit. Using your full range of motion is also better for injury prevention. You won't develop strength unevenly but rather throughout the entire movement pattern.

Good exercise form is equally crucial. Your body will always find ways to get the weight up but that doesn't mean that those ways are good for muscle development or your health. For example, beginners will often get on their toes at the end of an overhead press, which can be dangerous because it jeopardises their balance. This seems strange before you realize that what they have asked their body to do is to lift the weight as high as possible, using any means necessary. The body obeys and tries to gain extra height by lifting them on their toes. You need to be mindful of these things. It takes time to learn good exercise form and hiring a personal trainer is a good idea. If you don't want to hire a personal trainer, study each exercise from Youtube before you head out. Film yourself doing the exercise and identify where your form breaks down. Address these issues before problems arise.

With all that in mind your programming might look like this:

Month 1: Strength

- 3 full body workouts per week
- 1-5 rep range, 3-5 minute rest periods
- Focus on moving heavy weights but with good form and control

Exercise selection for month 1:

- Warm-up session focusing on creating good mind muscle connection and full range of motion
- One leg exercise such as squat, deadlift or lunge
- One pushing exercise such as bench press or overhead press
- One pulling exercise such as pull-up or barbell row
- One core exercise such as hanging leg raises or some sort of lever variation

Month 2: Muscle Growth

- 3 full body workouts per week
- 8-12 rep range, 60-90 second rest periods
- Focus on full range of motion and good muscle burn

Exercise selection for month 2:
- Warm-up session focusing on creating good mind muscle connection and full range of motion
- One leg exercise such as squat, deadlift (6 reps max) or lunge
- One pushing exercise such as bench dumbbell press or overhead dumbbell press
- One pulling exercise such as pull-up or dumbbell row
- One core exercise such as hanging leg raises or side chops

Month 3: Muscle Pump

- 3 full body workouts per week
- 12-20 rep range, 30-60 second rest periods
- Focus on full range of motion and extreme muscle burn

Exercise selection for month 3:
- Warm-up session focusing on creating good mind muscle connection and full range of motion
- One leg exercise such as squat or lunge
- One pushing exercise such as bench dumbbell press or

overhead dumbbell press
- One pulling exercise such as cable or dumbbell rows
- One cable exercise for additional bicep, tricep and shoulder growth
- One core exercise such as hanging leg raises or side chops

Month 4: Power

- 3 full body workouts per week
- 1-5 rep range, 3-5 minute rest periods
- Focus on explosive fast movement with good form and control

Exercise selection for month 4:
- Warm-up session focusing on creating good mind muscle connection and full range of motion
- One leg exercise such as squat, deadlift or lunge
- One pushing exercise such as bench press or overhead press
- One pulling exercise such as pull-up, barbell row or clean
- One core exercise such as hanging leg raises or some sort of lever variation

Then rotate back to month 1. Rinse and repeat. Every now and then take it easy for a few extra days.

Exercise Programming For Beginners

If you have never worked out before, I again strongly encourage you to start with 5x5 Stronglifts. It's simple and effective. It'll teach you all the important big lifts such as squats, deadlifts, bench and overhead presses and rows and it's a great mixture of strength and muscle size for a beginner. Google it, or get the free app and follow the instructions.

5x5 Stronglifts program

- 2 or 3 days a week
- Rotate between workout A and workout B

Workout A
- Squat, bench press and barbell row
- 5 sets of 5 reps per exercise with 2-3 minute rest in between

Workout B
- Squat, deadlift and overhead press
- 5 sets of 5 reps with squat and overhead press and 1 set of 5 reps of deadlift with 2-3 minute rest in between

After a few months when you're getting good at the lifts and getting stronger, it might be time to then graduate to a more complicated program like the one outlined above.

Study link:

https://www.ncbi.nlm.nih.gov/pubmed/11782267

REST, RECOVERY AND TRACKING

Managing your rest and recovery is as important as working out. If you're not fully rested when you work out, you're probably not making any progress. You're just burning yourself out. Here's a good rule of thumb: You should be stronger every time you go to the gym. If you're not stronger than last time, something's wrong. You haven't fully recovered from your last workout or you've been going after that same adaptation for too long and your body has stopped responding. If you don't track your workouts, you're not going to know this. Use pen and paper or since we're already living in the future, get an app and use that. I personally use one called Strong, which is great.

When you're tracking your workouts, you'll know if you're making progress or not. And if not, that's a sign that something is off. Are you eating enough? Getting good sleep? Do you feel stressed? Tools like the aforementioned Oura Ring can be very valuable in figuring this out. If you're going through a stressful period, maybe cut training back to 2 days a week from 3. Or use lighter weights for awhile. Practice the skills, take your time and don't go full beast mode. Sometimes less is more. Minimum effective dose to elicit the maximum amount of gains, remember?

Because working out is stressful, the first priority after a workout is to get out of that high-cortisol state. Try to relax and bring your heart rate down. Breathe deep. Listen to relaxing music instead of your heavy metal workout mix. Don't have coffee after a workout. Your stress-dose for the day is now done and the rest of the day should be as calm and peaceful as possible. Gains are made when you are zen.

All stress will affect your central nervous system and if the amplifier is not running smoothly, the speakers meaning your muscles will not work as they should. You can't train your way out of an overstressed CNS, rest and recovery is the only way to get your performance back. Managing your stress and sleep is even more important for someone who trains hard than it is for the Average Joe. Don't neglect them.

GETTING SHREDDED

By now we've covered how to get bigger and stronger, so let's move on to the next topic: Getting shredded. This vague term generally refers to getting to a low enough body fat where your muscles are clearly visible. You've got a six pack, defined shoulders, chest and back and probably some visible veins. For guys this means getting to less than 10% body fat. For women it's somewhere in the 12-18% range. Please note that nobody "needs" to be shredded. Healthy body fat range is pretty broad and when you start getting really low, you actually start to become less healthy. But it's fun to get shredded for the summer so what the hell, let's do it.

I'm sure you've read the fat loss chapter, right? If not, go back, do your homework and then come back. Same fundamental principles will apply. Creating an aesthetic athletic physique requires alternating between bulking and cutting. Sometimes you're bulking and focusing on growth, sometimes cutting down a bit. Cutting down equals fat burning. You're not trying to get rid of your muscles. Note that going through phases of bulking and cutting is beneficial for anyone. If you're not trying to get to a very low body fat percentage, just keep the cuts short. Cutting and bulking will prevent the body from getting too used to any single calorie level. After every cut, when you go for a bulk, you'll be more anabolic because of elevated growth hormone levels.

Bulking and cutting essentially means undulating your calories from high to low. You shouldn't stay in one modality for too long. If you're always trying to bulk, your body will get used to the high calorie intake and will speed up your metabolism. You're eating more but you're also burning more calories and it gets harder and harder to keep upping the ante. Similarly if you cut for too long, your metabolism will slow down and your body will start to cannibalise muscle because it's trying to create a slower metabolism. To avoid these pitfalls, keep the bulks and cuts short. Less than a month, ideally even shorter. A good rule of thumb is to up your calories 500 kcal a day when bulking and drop them 500 when cutting. But since we're not fans of counting calories here, let's just say that the difference is one meal per day. When bulking, eat one more meal. When cutting, eat one less.

Stay mindful of your workouts when bulking or cutting. Bulking obviously is very well suited for building muscle and strength. Cutting is not. So during a cut don't worry about the results in the gym so much. You're not trying to build muscle right now. You're trying to maintain it. The reason you work out during a cut is to keep sending those anabolic signals via testosterone and growth hormone and reminding the body that getting rid of muscle is not an option. A great way to increase your fat-burning while cutting is to get more active outside the gym. Walk more than usual, take a yoga class or you might even*GASP* go for a jog every now and then.

When cutting, working out on an empty stomach can be very effective. When the body doesn't have lots of energy stores available in the gut, it will be forced to mobilize some fat to fuel your needs. Even if you usually like to work out in the evenings, try shifting it to the early morning or around noon when you're cutting.

Intermittent fasting is especially great when it comes to cutting. Since you'll be skipping one meal per day in a cutting phase anyway, try to shrink your feeding window down. If previously you were practicing the 16 hour fast / 8 hour feeding window -system, try going to 18/6 or even 20/4 every now and then.

With these practices you'll be setting the stage for an optimal anabolic environment and truly becoming a fat burning beast. Just keep in mind that fasting is another stressor for the body. It's a powerful tool and all power tools need to be used with caution.

BUT I JUST WANT TO LOOK LIKE BRAD PITT IN FIGHT CLUB

Yeah so do I. Brad looked amazing. So you should then just google "Brad Pitt Fight Club workout" and follow that, right? No. You're not Brad Pitt. And that's why you won't look like Brad Pitt even if you followed the same exact exercise program and diet. We don't know if Brad got shredded for the role all naturally without anabolic steroids but even if he did, his genetics and natural hormone levels are different from yours and mine. And we don't get paid millions to work out for months and months with the help of personal trainers, with professional chefs cooking our every meal with perfect macronutrient distribution. We got jobs and kids, and you know, a life.

And since we're on the topic of celebrities and other fitness influencers, let's stay there for a bit. It's getting more and more common for the fit & beautiful Instagram-famous guys and gals to sell their personal top secret diet and exercise programs that are guaranteed to get everyone into the same shape as they are. This is complete and utter bullcrap. People are different and what worked for them won't work with everyone. In addition, these people usually aren't experts in health and fitness, they are experts in posing and looking good in photos. We all knew people growing up who always looked handsome and beautiful. Would you take their advice on how to become beautiful? No because they wouldn't know the first thing about how to become beautiful. It just happened to them. Same story with these celebrities. They just know how they got to where they are. They don't know a thing about you.

Don't get duped by marketing gimmicks. You can get into an amazing shape, but your amazing shape will look different from mine and Brad Pitt's. And that's a good thing. There are no shortcuts in health & fitness.

CHEAT DAYS AND LETTING LOOSE

It also seems like every Instagram fitness influencer loves to talk about their cheat days. I hate this concept. Having a cheat day implies that you're somehow depriving yourself of something every other day. It reinforces a very poor relationship to health, exercise and diet. It feeds body image issues and mental health problems such as anorexia or bulimia. Don't have cheat days. Every now and then you'll probably have more carbs, alcohol, stay up late or whatever your vice might be. Don't make a big deal about it.

Most everyday people who have fitness goals still tend to let loose on the weekends. They work hard and stay regimented during the week, then drink, party and eat whatever comes to mind during the weekend. If this is what you want, no problem. Enjoy life the way you want. But if you're struggling to reach your goals, consider the following: Let's say every time you work out, eat right or get good sleep, you get plus points. Every time you drink alcohol, get poor sleep and eat unhealthy foods, you get minus points. More plus points, more muscle gains. More minus points, you're sabotaging your progress. Intuitively thinking, taking 2 or 3 days off from a 7 day week doesn't feel like much. But you're not only missing out on the plus points you could have compiled during the weekend, you're also accruing lots of minus points. Here's an example:

Monday: workout, healthy eating, good sleep. **3 plus points**
Tuesday: healthy eating, good sleep: **2 plus points (total 5)**

Wednesday: healthy eating, good sleep: **2 plus points (total 7)**

Thursday: workout, healthy eating, good sleep. **3 plus points (total 10)**

Friday: unhealthy eating, alcohol, poor sleep. **3 minus points (total 7)**

Saturday: workout, unhealthy eating, alcohol, poor sleep. **1 plus point and 3 minus points (total 5)**

Sunday: unhealthy eating, good sleep. 1 plus point, 1 minus point. **(Total 5)**

According to this model you essentially sabotaged all the progress you made after tuesday. Had you stayed on track during the weekend you'd be at 18 points. Over 3 times better than the 5 where you wound up. Now of course this is just a hypothetical example, not exactly how life works. But it beautifully illustrates the point. Whenever you do anything, there will be consequences. Think about your priorities and make your lifestyle choices based on them.

LIFESTYLE HABITS FOR CORRECT HORMONAL BALANCE

By now I'm sure you've got a pretty good read on things. There's no need to repeat basics like getting good sleep, managing your stress, eating real whole foods and staying active. See what I did there? These basic fundamental things are worth repeating endlessly and endlessly.

It's way too easy to start slipping when you're making progress and feeling good. But over time those extra cups of coffee at work, staying up later than normal, alcohol here and there and eating more processed foods and so on will start to add up. Your progress will slow down, halt or even reverse. And digging yourself out of a hole is a whole lot more difficult than avoiding falling into the hole to begin with.

Healthy lifestyle habits are more important for someone who works out regularly, not less. Your baseline level of stress is higher than of a couch potato. You just might not feel it because of the hormones and other feel good -chemicals from all that exercise are keeping you going. Remember: Cortisol kills testosterone. Keep working out but also work in: Meditate, do yoga, take walks, enjoy the moment and be grateful for your progress. Respect your sleep schedule above all else.

SUPPLEMENTS

Yes, there is one supplement you probably should take: creatine. As you remember, your body generates those first few seconds of power and strength through the creatine-phosphocreatine pathway and if you're supplementing with creatine, you'll have more gas in the tank. Now, supplemental creatine is still not going to make a huge difference, especially if you're not vegan or vegetarian. For vegans it might make a big difference because you mainly get your creatine through meat and thus vegans might be deficient. The studies on creatine do tend to show a consistent moderate increase in strength, so I'd say it's worth the money. And it's dirt cheap by the way. Just get standard creatine monohydrate and use 5 grams every day. One study did show that it was most effective when taken after a workout. But take it when it's most convenient to you.

There are a couple of downsides to creatine though: If you're a man, it might speed up male pattern baldness (if you already got it) because it'll increase conversion of testosterone to dihydrotestosterone (DHT). In terms of strength and performance, there's nothing wrong with this but higher levels of DHT have been linked to speeding up hair loss. Creatine will also make you hold on to more water which might make you look a bit puffier (or bigger) than usual. And it's also been linked to acne, but that seems to be pretty rare. With these caveats in mind, it's a good supplement.

There are a gazillion strength building supplements on the market and some of them do work. But again, lift the big rocks first. If you've been working out years and are doing everything else right, then it might be fun to mess around with supplements. Just be prepared to spend lots of money and get disappointed often.

As mentioned in the weight loss chapter, addressing nutritional deficiencies can be very useful. If you're eating a wide variety of whole foods and your gut health is good, you're on the right track but you still might have some blind spots. There are some nutrients that are strongly linked to the anabolic hormones: For example zinc status plays a big part in testosterone. So for example eat some oysters every now and then. And if your cholesterol is low, you'll have a hard time making testosterone. Have some cholesterol-rich meals after your workout: Whole eggs are the bomb.

But this is all the type of nitty gritty stuff you should only get into after awhile of doing all the right things. Don't worry about it too much. Remember how in the beginning we talked about how the body is stronger than the sum of its parts. With all the healthy lifestyle habits you're now following, you're making it more and more resilient every day.

Study links:

https://www.ncbi.nlm.nih.gov/pubmed/?term=creatine +strength

https://www.ncbi.nlm.nih.gov/pubmed/23919405

TIPS AND TROUBLESHOOTING

Don't even read this section before you have your bases covered. Nothing else will give you the same benefits as good sleep, smart exercise programming and hormone-friendly lifestyle. But if you're already doing everything we talked about and would want to see more progress, there might be a couple of things to address.

How Do I Know Where I Stand

So you've been following the advice of the book for awhile and are not sure if it's all working. Ask yourself a few things: How do you feel? How do you perform? How do you look? If the answer to all these things is "better", you're on the right path. Keep doing what you're doing. If the answer is not "better", try switching things around. Eat cleaner, have more or less carbs, increase or decrease your protein intake, increase or decrease your exercise volume, go out in the sun, take holidays and definitely make sleep a priority. Some hormonal results are also pretty easy to feel. If you feel stressed, it means your cortisol is going up. If you're a man and wake up with morning wood, your testosterone is going up. Regardless of whether you're a man or a woman, if your sex drive is increasing, testosterone and growth hormone are going up.

If you just don't know, consider getting some lab tests done. Human growth hormone and testosterone are interlinked so there's really no need to measure growth hormone, which is a very tricky hormone to measure anyway. But get a basic testosterone panel.

Total And Free Testosterone

If you're a man and get your testosterone test done in in a lab, they'll usually measure 3 things: total testosterone, free testosterone and Sex hormone binding globulin or SHBG for short. Essentially if your body is producing 1000 units of testosterone, only some of it will be so called free testosterone, which is the bioavailable physiologically active form, used by the body. Some will be hijacked on the way by SHBG which as the name implies, binds to sex hormones such as testosterone and estrogen. If your SHBG is very high, your free testosterone might be low even if your body is producing a lot of testosterone. I had this problem, and most likely the reason was my jeopardized gut health. Reasons for high SHBG aren't always very clear but SHBG does also naturally go up with age. It also seems to go up with infections and other inflammatory conditions. And my gut was definitely inflamed for a long time. However, since then, I've more than doubled my free testosterone and my SHBG has dropped to normal levels by following the advice layed out in this book.

First of all, before you do anything, measure your testosterone. Note that testosterone is highly fluctuable and if you for example had poor sleep the night before the test, you'll get a lower result. So don't freak out regardless of the result. If your SHBG is low but your total and free testosterone are still low, double down on the advice given in this book. You'll get it up. However, if your SHBG is high, you might want to consider some additional things

Fixing Your Shbg And Testosterone Levels

Most likely the reason behind your high SHBG is inflammatory, so again take extra steps with your diet, sleep and stress management. You need to first heal yourself for your SHBG to lower. If you have gut problems, try longer fasts as mentioned in the weight loss chapter. Try going keto or conversely upping your carbs if you've been low carb previously. Gut problems will also contribute to nutritional deficiencies so it's worth supplementing with some of the most important co-factors. Most important minerals for testosterone production are zinc and magnesium but interestingly boron seems to be a good mineral in lowering SHBG. Try supplementing with zinc, magnesium and boron. Only choose good reputable brands. Cheap chinese made supplements are known to contain all kinds of garbage and might not even have the minerals you're looking for.

Plastics, and the xenoestrogens found in them will also hurt your testosterone levels. Avoid eating and drinking from plastic containers. Only use natural skin care products. A good rule of thumb with any skin care product is this: Would you eat it? If you wouldn't eat it, why would you let your body absorb it through the skin? Don't go crazy, but stay mindful of what you're putting into your body. Saunas are great for increasing detoxification of toxic and unwanted substances through sweating.

Test Again

After you've switched some things around, healed your gut, supplemented with the right minerals and whatever else you might have done, it's time to take the test again. Wait at least 6 months between the tests though and again, be mindful that the results will fluctuate heavily based on life stress. Don't go after a deadlift personal record the previous day before a testosterone test. Regardless of the numbers, go by how you feel. If you feel good, it doesn't really matter what the numbers look like.

Different bodies will also utilize testosterone differently. If you have lots of testosterone receptors, you're very sensitive to testosterone and need less of it. And vice versa, some people might need high amounts of testosterone because like with all the other hormones, bodies can become resistant to them.

CLOSING WORDS

Remember that hormones alone can make a bigger impact on your muscle gains than exercising. Respect this fact and take care of your hormones first, even if it means sacrificing workouts for better recovery.

It's always hard to start working out. Once you start to see progress, it's hard to stop. Keep doing the right things and let this momentum carry you forward. Willpower to get to the gym is the only thing really needed at the beginning. After a few months, you'll need some of that willpower to pull back and not work too hard. Enjoy this new balance you've created.

Stay anabolic my friends.

P.S. But not all the time.

CHAPTER 5: RESOURCES AND RECOMMENDATIONS

Chances are you got further interested in some topic while reading this book and would like to dive a little bit deeper. In this chapter I've outlined some books, websites and podcasts that are great on any specific topic.

Sleep

Why We Sleep: Unlocking the Power of Sleep and Dreams by Matthew Walker

A great read on the biology of sleep, and the consequences of good and bad sleep.

Diet

Books:

The Keto Reset Diet: Reboot Your Metabolism in 21 Days and Burn Fat Forever by Mark Sisson

Mark Sisson is "the godfather of paleo" and his website Mark's Daily Apple has long been one of my favorites. The Keto Reset Diet is a great book. Don't be alarmed by the cheesy name. It thoroughly explains the benefits and potential downsides of "going keto", ie starting a ketogenic diet.

Wired to Eat: Turn Off Cravings, Rewire Your Appetite for Weight Loss, and Determine the Foods That Work for You by Robb Wolf

If Mark Sisson is the godfather of the paleo movement, Robb Wolf is at least the godson. Wired to Eat explains in great detail how and why we overeat and what to do about it.

The Longevity Diet: Discover the New Science Behind Stem Cell Activation and Regeneration to Slow Aging, Fight Disease, and Optimize Weight by Dr. Valter Longo

A great book by Valter Longo that explains the benefits of fasting and introduces Valter's Fasting Mimicking Diet. The author has been studying fasting for a long time and the science in the book is very solid.

Healthy Gut, Healthy You: The Personalized Plan to Transform Your Health from the Inside Out by Dr. Michael Ruscio

A great book on gut health with a very actionable plan in creating your individual diet for better gut health.

Fat for Fuel: A Revolutionary Diet to Combat Cancer, Boost Brain Power, and Increase Your Energy by Dr. Joseph Mercola

A very solid read despite the hyperbolic title. Explains to the reader how a ketogenic diet can be an extremely healthy diet in several ways.

Other media:

The Paleo Solution podcast

Pretty self-explanatory as the name suggests. Robb Wolf's podcast where he answers listener questions and interviews all kinds of people

FoundMyFitness podcast

Dr Rhonda Patrick's podcast which is insanely interesting for geeks such as myself. Rhonda dives deep on several topics and includes study links and other useful resources to each episode.

Ben Greenfield Fitness

Ben Greenfield is a weird man, and that's what makes him interesting. A biohacker who's willing to try anything to optimize his performance, be it physical or mental.

Stress

Buddha's Brain: The Practical Neuroscience of Happiness, Love, and Wisdom by Rick Hanson

Basic mindfulness and meditation techniques explained through the lens of modern neuroscience. A great read with very practical examples and exercises.

Movement

Books:

Becoming a Supple Leopard: The Ultimate Guide to Resolving Pain, Preventing Injury, and Optimizing Athletic Performance by Kelly Starrett

A true bible of the human body. Kelly explains in great detail how different muscle groups work with any major lift and goes into detail on rehab strategies and maintaining good performance.

Move Your DNA: Restore Your Health Through Natural Movement by Katy Bowman

A great book on the physical benefits of being uncomfortable, be it sleeping on a hard mattress or walking barefoot.

Other media:

The MindPump podcast

A hilarious but highly informative podcast where 3 personal trainers teach the fundamentals of exercise and diet for body composition changes.

Posture: the Key to Good Health | Annette Verpillot | TEDxMontreal Women

This is a TedX video you can find on Youtube. It can be a life changing experience if you have any tightness or pain issues. Annette shows a simple eye tracking exercise which might just be the most powerful pain alleviating tool I've ever encountered.

Technology And Apps

Here are my recommendations on different fitness and diet technology and apps:

The Oura Ring

My fitness tracker of choice. The Oura measures everything from movement to sleep and heart rate variability. And it's just a ring, no need to wear a bulky watch on your wrist all the time.

Strong

A great app to track your workouts.

Stronglifts

Another great fitness app for tracking your 5x5 Stronglifts workouts.

FatSecret

Good app for calculating the macronutrient content of a meal.

Cara

Another useful app for trying to find what diet works for you. You keep track of what you eat and how you feel and Cara will show you which foods are most likely to cause problems for you.

Brain.fm

Weirdly great app for relaxation and focus. Brain.fm creates music that "tunes" your brain to a specific mood, be it about focus or relaxation or sleep. I've used the focus-mode in writing this book quite often. At least for me it works great.

What did you think of 'Hormone Optimization' ?

First of all my sincerest thanks for purchasing and reading this book. You could have picked any number of books to read on the subject but you chose this one and I am extremely grateful. I hope this book provided value to your everyday life and gave you some concrete tools to get you closer to your goals.

If you enjoyed this book and it provided you with some benefit, I'd like to hear from you and hope that you could take some time to post a review on Amazon. Your feedback and support will greatly help the writer improve his writing craft and make future versions of this book even better.

My sincerest thanks,
Joonas